Collected
WRITINGS

LOUIS PASTEUR
AND JOSEPH LISTER

FOREWORD BY
DR. CONRAD FISCHER

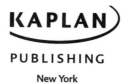

KAPLAN

PUBLISHING

New York

Foreword by Dr. Conrad Fischer © 2008

Published by Kaplan Publishing, a division of Kaplan, Inc.
1 Liberty Plaza, 24th Floor
New York, NY 10006

Printed in the United States of America

August 2008

10 9 8 7 6 5 4 3 2 1

ISBN-13: 978-1-4277-9800-8

Kaplan Publishing books are available at special quantity discounts to use for sales promotions, employee premiums, or educational purposes. Please email our Special Sales Department to order or for more information at kaplanpublishing@kaplan.com, or write to Kaplan Publishing, 1 Liberty Plaza, 24th Floor, New York, NY 10006.

CONTENTS

FOREWORD

"Where observation is concerned, chance favors only the prepared mind."

—Louis Pasteur

One day in 1885, a rapid dog ran loose in the streets of Newark, New Jersey. The dog mauled six children before it was killed. Devastated parents awaited the first sign of rabies: hydrophobia, the compulsive, involuntary fear of water. Imagine your child delirious with thirst but unable to drink and doomed to die a few days or weeks later—no treatment, no hope! Then, word reached the city of a scientist in France who had developed a method to treat and prevent this abomination. The children might be spared the alternate method of treatment: searing the wounds with a red hot iron. Donations poured in from common people and philanthropists. Four children boarded a ship for France. They were treated in Paris with a new method called vaccination, given progressively stronger doses of injections of dried rabbit spinal cord tissue.

One month later, four healthy children returned to Newark. Their savior, Dr. Louis Pasteur, chemist and supreme advocate of the experimental method, triumphed when all hope seemed lost.

Louis Pasteur achieved remarkable discoveries in microbiology than would now only be expected in the lifetimes of a dozen scientists. Some of his discoveries were the results of purposeful, planned investigation. Some were successful by accident. Yet no matter the origin of his accomplishments, Pasteur's glory lay in the innumerable lives that his results saved. As a scientist, his aim was no less than to "lift up a corner of the veil behind which God has hidden the secrets of the universe."

Pasteur rose to fame by lending his genius to the most French of French endeavors. Winemakers (and scientists) debated whether fermentation was simply a chemical process or the result of a microorganism. In 1860, France and the United Kingdom signed a free-trade agreement. In anticipation of an explosion of wine exports to England, merchants and farmers asked Pasteur to investigate why wine turns sour.

In a restaurant, the waiter pours a little taste of wine for you to see if it is sour. It almost never is. Yet, during the 19th century, sour wine was common. Pasteur used his microscope and experimental observational talents to determine that although yeast may produce alcohol from fermentation, it is the proliferation of bacteria that makes it sour. Pasteur discovered that if the wine was heated briefly to 50–60 degrees centigrade, it did not spoil. *Oh no!* cried his detractors. *Pasteur will 'cook' our wine and ruin its taste! Disgusting!*

To counter this argument, Pasteur gathered a panel of judges to taste both the heated and the unheated wine. The heated wine won the taste test, and we were on our way to a better glass of wine. Pasteur's results led him to explore whether microorganisms could also infect humans. It was these experiments in fermentation that led to his germ theory, which you are about to read. Alas, during his most notable experiments, Pasteur's 12-year-old daughter Cecille came down with a fever. Within two weeks she died of typhoid, a microorganism now known as *Salmonella typhi*. Eventually Pasteur definitively disproved the idea of "spontaneous generation," the belief that organisms can arise out of nothing in decaying matter, but too late to save his own child.

During the height of Pasteur's career, a brilliant surgeon in Scotland was examining his medical records. Despite the best practices of the time, 50% of all his amputation cases had died of infection between 1861 and 1865. The surgeon's name was Joseph Lister, and in 1865, he read of Pasteur's germ theory and became determined to eliminate microorganisms from the operative field. Lister noticed that workers in his native Edinburgh sprayed carbolic acid, a derivative of coal tar, into the city sewage to eliminate the foul smell of decay. Lister immediately insisted that all his instruments be washed with carbolic acid. He stopped repeatedly during operations to rinse his hands in the same liquid. He covered wounds with a dressing drenched in carbolic acid and packed them with a putty infused with carbolic acid. He even went so far as to insist on spraying the acid into the air of the operating theater. The nurses and staff barely tolerated the eccentricities of this surgeon who believed in funny little bugs that no one can see that invaded wounds to cause infection, sepsis, and death. After all, 'hospitalism'—a phrase describing the gangrene condition that resulted in half of all surgical patients—was a common phenomenon. But no one argued with Lister's results: within two years, operative mortality decreased from nearly 50% to just 15%.

By Lister's death in 1912, the death rate from amputation had fallen to 3%. His discoveries surely saved the lives of untold thousands during the First World War.

Lister also developed catgut, the first sterile, dissolvable suture material. Despite its name, catgut was derived from the sheep intestines and could be easily sterilized to prevent infection. Still, in response to this momentous achievement, the medical world did what it did best in that era: ignored or rejected Lister's idea. After all, few physicians can bear the idea that their 'best practices' are killing their patients.

But Lister was not alone in meeting skepticism. In 1879, a presenter at the Academy of Medicine in Paris described "childbed fever" as a metabolic disease. But a voice from the audience interrupted, shouting, "None of these things cause the epidemic; it is the nursing and medical staff who carry the microbe from an infected woman to a healthy one." That voice belonged to Pasteur.

Much of the greatness of Pasteur and Lister lies in their dogged persistence to spend 20 years convincing the rest of the medical world of the truth of their investigations. They are frustrated, yes, angry, yes, but they persist, and they prevail.

In this volume, you will find the original words of these courageous and brilliant men. In a society with many celebrities, but few heroes, it is a joy for us to journey to the past and imagine their accomplishments within the context of their times.

What is the invisible plague of our era? Is it depression that leads to 1,000 deaths per week from suicide? Is it AIDS or cancer? Or is it malaria, which still kills 2 million people per year, half of whom are children, with no vaccine in sight?

Read on and ponder who among us will be the next Pasteur or Lister. Someone, we hope, will not only discover a cure, but also have the strength of character to persuade a world that still hasn't learned to wash its hands.

Dr. Conrad Fischer
April, 2008

"The life of a scientist is so short! So numerous are the mysteries of nature, especially of living nature"

—Louis Pasteur

GERM THEORY AND ITS APPLICATIONS TO MEDICINE AND SURGERY

Louis Pasteur

The Sciences gain by mutual support. When, as the result of my first communications on the fermentations in 1857–1858, it appeared that the ferments, properly so-called, are living beings, that the germs of microscopic organisms abound in the surface of all objects, in the air and in water; that the theory of spontaneous generation is chimerical; that wines, beer, vinegar, the blood, urine and all the fluids of the body undergo none of their usual changes in pure air, both Medicine and Surgery received fresh stimulation. A French physician, Dr. Davaine, was fortunate in making the first application of these principles to Medicine, in 1863.

Our researches of last year, left the etiology of the putrid disease, or septicemia, in a much less advanced condition than that of anthrax. We had demonstrated the probability that septicemia depends upon the presence and growth of a microscopic body, but the absolute proof of this important conclusion was not reached. To demonstrate experimentally that a microscopic organism actually is the cause of a disease and the agent of contagion, I know no other way, in the present state of Science, than to subject the microbe (the new and happy term introduced by

M. Sedillot) to the method of cultivation out of the body. It may be noted that in twelve successive cultures, each one of only ten cubic centimeters volume, the original drop will be diluted as if placed in a volume of fluid equal to the total volume of the earth. It is just this form of test to which M. Joubert and I subjected the anthrax bacteridium.[2] Having cultivated it a great number of times in a sterile fluid, each culture being started with a minute drop from the preceding, we then demonstrated that the product of the last culture was capable of further development and of acting in the animal tissues by producing anthrax with all its symptoms. Such is—as we believe—the indisputable proof that anthrax is a bacterial disease.

Our researches concerning the septic vibrio had not so far been convincing, and it was to fill up this gap that we resumed our experiments. To this end, we attempted the cultivation of the septic vibrio from an animal dead of septicemia. It is worth noting that all of our first experiments failed, despite the variety of culture media we employed—urine, beer yeast water, meat water, etc. Our culture media were not sterile, but we found most commonly—a microscopic organism showing no relationship to the septic vibrio, and presenting the form, common enough elsewhere, of chains of extremely minute spherical granules possessed of no virulence whatever.[3] This was an impurity, introduced, unknown to us, at the same time as the septic vibrio; and the germ undoubtedly passed from the intestines—always inflamed and distended in septicemic animals—into the abdominal fluids from which we took our original cultures of the septic

[2] In making the translation, it seems wiser to adhere to Pasteur's nomenclature. Bacillus anthracis would be the term employed to-day. Translator.

[3] It is quite possible that Pasteur was here dealing with certain septicemic streptococci that are now known to lose their virulence with extreme rapidity under artificial cultivation.—Translator.

vibrio. If this explanation of the contamination of our cultures was correct, we ought to find a pure culture of the septic vibrio in the heart's blood of an animal recently dead of septicemia. This was what happened, but a new difficulty presented itself; all our cultures remained sterile. Furthermore this sterility was accompanied by loss in the culture media of (the original) virulence.

It occurred to us that the septic vibrio might be an obligatory anaerobe and that the sterility of our inoculated culture fluids might be due to the destruction of the septic vibrio by the atmospheric oxygen dissolved in the fluids. The Academy may remember that I have previously demonstrated facts of this nature in regard to the vibrio of butyric fermentation, which not only lives without air but is killed by the air.

It was necessary therefore to attempt to cultivate the septic vibrio either in a vacuum or in the presence of inert gases—such as carbonic acid.

Results justified our attempt; the septic vibrio grew easily in a complete vacuum, and no less easily in the presence of pure carbonic acid.

These results have a necessary corollary. If a fluid containing septic vibrios be exposed to pure air, the vibrios should be killed and all virulence should disappear. This is actually the case. If some drops of septic serum be spread horizontally in a tube and in a very thin layer, the fluid will become absolutely harmless in less than half a day, even if at first it was so virulent as to produce death upon the inoculation of the smallest portion of a drop.

Furthermore all the vibrios, which crowded the liquid as motile threads, are destroyed and disappear. After the action of the air, only fine amorphous granules can be found, unfit for culture as well as for the transmission of any disease whatever. It might be said that the air burned the vibrios.

If it is a terrifying thought that life is at the mercy of the multiplication of these minute bodies, it is a consoling hope that Science will not always remain powerless before such enemies, since for example at the very beginning of the study we find that simple exposure to air is sufficient at times to destroy them.

But, if oxygen destroys the vibrios, how can septicemia exist, since atmospheric air is present everywhere? How can such facts be brought in accord with the germ theory? How can blood, exposed to air, become septic through the dust the air contains?

All things are hidden, obscure and debatable if the cause of the phenomena be unknown, but everything is clear if this cause be known. What we have just said is true only of a septic fluid containing adult vibrios, in active development by fission: conditions are different when the vibrios are transformed into their germs,[4] that is into the glistening corpuscles first described and figured in my studies on silk-worm disease, in dealing with worms dead of the disease called "flacherie." Only the adult vibrios disappear, burn up, and lose their virulence in contact with air: the germ corpuscles, under these conditions, remain always ready for new cultures, and for new inoculations.

All this however does not do away with the difficulty of understanding how septic germs can exist on the surface of objects, floating in the air and in water.

Where can these corpuscles originate? Nothing is easier than the production of these germs, in spite of the presence of air in contact with septic fluids.

[4] By the terms "germ" and "germ corpuscles," Pasteur undoubtedly means "spores," but the change is not made, in accordance with note 2,—Translator.

If abdominal serous exudate containing septic vibrios actively growing by fission be exposed to the air, as we suggested above, but with the precaution of giving a substantial thickness to the layer, even if only one centimeter be used, this curious phenomenon will appear in a few hours. The oxygen is absorbed in the upper layers of the fluid—as is indicated by the change of color. Here the vibrios are dead and disappear. In the deeper layers, on the other hand, towards the bottom of this centimeter of septic fluid we suppose to be under observation, the vibrios continue to multiply by fission-protected from the action of oxygen by those that have perished above them: little by little they pass over to the condition of germ corpuscles with the gradual disappearance of the thread forms. So that instead of moving threads of varying length, sometimes greater than the field of the microscope, there is to be seen only a number of glittering points, lying free or surrounded by a scarcely perceptible amorphous mass.[5] Thus is formed, containing the latent germ life, no longer in danger from the destructive action of oxygen, thus, I repeat, is formed the septic dust, and we are able to understand what has before seemed so obscure; we can see how putrescible fluids can be inoculated by the dust of the air, and how it is that putrid diseases are permanent in the world.

The Academy will permit me, before leaving these interesting results, to refer to one of their main theoretical consequences. At the very beginning of these researches, for they reveal an entirely new field, what must be insistently demanded? The

[5] In our note of July 16th, 1877, it is stated that the septic vibrio is not destroyed by the oxygen of the air nor by oxygen at high tension, but that under these conditions it is transformed into germ corpuscles. This is, however, an incorrect interpretation of facts. The vibrio is destroyed by oxygen, and it is only where it is in a thick layer that it is transformed to germ-corpuscles in the presence of oxygen and that its virulence is preserved.

absolute proof that there actually exist transmissible, contagious, infectious diseases of which the cause lies essentially and solely in the presence of microscopic organisms. The proof that for at least some diseases, the conception of spontaneous virulence must be forever abandoned—as well as the idea of contagion and an infectious element suddenly originating in the bodies of men or animals and able to originate diseases which propagate themselves under identical forms: and all of those opinions fatal to medical progress, which have given rise to the gratuitous hypotheses of spontaneous generation, of albuminoid ferments, of hemiorganisms, of archebiosis, and many other conceptions without the least basis in observation. What is to be sought for in this instance is the proof that along with our vibrio there does not exist an independent virulence belonging to the surrounding fluids or solids, in short that the vibrio is not merely an epiphenomenon of the disease of which it is the obligatory accompaniment. What then do we see, in the results that I have just brought out? A septic fluid, taken at the moment that the vibrios are not yet changed into germs, loses its virulence completely upon simple exposure to the air, but preserves this virulence, although exposed to air on the simple condition of being in a thick layer for some hours. In the first case, the virulence once lost by exposure to air, the liquid is incapable of taking it on again upon cultivation: but, in the second case, it preserves its virulence and can propagate, even after exposure to air. It is impossible, then, to assert that there is a separate virulent substance, either fluid or solid, existing, apart from the adult vibrio or its germ. Nor can it be supposed that there is a virus which loses its virulence at the moment that the adult vibrio dies; for such a substance should also lose its virulence when the vibrios, changed to germs, are exposed to the air. Since the virulence persists under these conditions it can only be due to the germ corpuscles—the only thing present. There is only one possible hypothesis as to the existence of a virus in solution, and that is that such a substance, which was present in our experiment in non-fatal amounts, should be continuously furnished by the vibrio itself, during its growth in the body of the living animal. But it is of little importance since the hypothesis supposes the forming and necessary existence of the vibrio.[6]

I hasten to touch upon another series of observations which are even more deserving the attention of the surgeon than the preceding: I desire to speak of the effects of our microbe of pus when associated with the septic vibrio. There is nothing more easy to superpose—as it were—two distinct diseases and to produce what might be called a septicemic purulent infection, or a purulent septicemia. Whilst the microbe-producing pus, when acting alone, gives rise to a thick pus, white, or sometimes with a yellow or bluish tint, not putrid, diffused or enclosed by the so-called pyogenic membrane, not dangerous, especially if localized in cellular tissue, ready, if the expression may be used for rapid resorption; on the other hand the smallest abscess produced by this organism when associated with the septic vibrio takes on a thick gangrenous appearance, putrid, greenish and infiltrating the softened tissues. In this case the microbe of pus carried so to speak by the septic vibrio, accompanies it throughout the body: the highly-inflamed muscular tissues, full of serous fluid, showing also globules of pus here and there, are like a kneading of the two organisms.

By a similar procedure the effects of the anthrax bacteridium and the microbe of pus may be combined and the two diseases may be superposed, so as to obtain a purulent anthrax or an

[6] The regular limits oblige me to omit a portion of my speech.

anthracoid purulent infection. Care must be taken not to exaggerate the predominance of the new microbe over the bacteridium. If the microbe be associated with the latter in sufficient amount it may crowd it out completely—prevent it from growing in the body at all. Anthrax does not appear, and the infection, entirely local, becomes merely an abscess whose cure is easy. The microbe-producing pus and the septic vibrio (not)[7] being both anaerobes, as we have demonstrated, it is evident that the latter will not much disturb its neighbor. Nutrient substances, fluid or solid, can scarcely be deficient in the tissues from such minute organisms. But the anthrax bacteridium is exclusively aerobic, and the proportion of oxygen is far from being equally distributed throughout the tissues: innumerable conditions can diminish or exhaust the supply here and there, and since the microbe-producing pus is also aerobic, it can be understood how, by using a quantity slightly greater than that of the bacteridium it might easily deprive the latter of the oxygen necessary for it. But the explanation of the fact is of little importance: it is certain that under some conditions the microbe we are speaking of entirely prevents the development of the bacteridium.

Summarizing—it appears from the preceding facts that it is possible to produce at will, purulent infections with no elements of putrescence, putrescent purulent infections, anthracoid purulent infections, and finally combinations of these types of lesions varying according to the proportions of the mixtures of the specific organisms made to act on the living tissues.

---

[7] There is undoubtedly a mistake in the original. Pasteur could not have meant to say that both bacteria are anaerobes. The word "not" is introduced to correct the error.—Translator.

These are the principal facts I have to communicate to the Academy in my name and in the names of my collaborators, Messrs. Joubert and Chamberland. Some weeks ago (Session of the 11th of March last) a member of the Section of Medicine and Surgery, M. Sedillot, after long meditation on the lessons of a brilliant career, did not hesitate to assert that the successes as well as the failures of Surgery find a rational explanation in the principles upon which the germ theory is based, and that this theory would found a new Surgery—already begun by a celebrated English surgeon, Dr. Lister,[8] who was among the first to understand its fertility. With no professional authority, but with the conviction of a trained experimenter, I venture here to repeat the words of an eminent confrere.

[8] In 1880. Especially engaged in the study of chicken cholera and the attenuation of virulence—Translator.

ON THE EXTENSION OF THE GERM THEORY TO THE ETIOLOGY OF CERTAIN COMMON DISEASES

When I began the studies now occupying my attention, I was attempting to extend the germ theory to certain common diseases. I do not know when I can return to that work. Therefore in my desire to see it carried on by others, I take the liberty of presenting it to the public in its present condition.

I. Furuncles.

In May, 1879, one of the workers in my laboratory had a number of furuncles, appearing at short intervals, sometimes on one part of the body and sometimes on another. Constantly impressed with the thought of the immense part played by microscopic organisms in Nature, I queried whether the pus in the furuncles might not contain one of these organisms whose presence, development, and chance transportation here and there in the tissues after entrance would produce a local inflammation, and pus formation, and might explain the recurrence of the illness during a longer or shorter time. It was easy enough to subject this thought to the test of experiment.

First observation.—On June second, a puncture was made at the base of the small cone of pus at the apex of a furuncle on the nape of the neck. The fluid obtained was at once sowed in the presence of pure air—of course with the precautions necessary to exclude any foreign germs, either at the moment of puncture, at the moment of sowing in the culture fluid, or during the stay in the oven, which was kept at the constant temperature of about 35 degrees C. The next day, the culture fluid had become cloudy and contained a single organism, consisting of small spherical points arranged in pairs, sometimes in fours, but often in irregular masses. Two fluids were preferred in these experiments—chicken and yeast bouillon. According as one or the other was used, appearances varied a little. These should be described. With the yeast water, the pairs of minute granules are distributed throughout the liquid, which is uniformly clouded. But with the chicken bouillon, the granules are collected in little masses which line the walls and bottom of the flasks while the body of the fluid remains clear, unless it be shaken: in this case it becomes uniformly clouded by the breaking up of the small masses from the walls of the flasks.

Second observation.—On the tenth of June a new furuncle made its appearance on the right thigh of the same person. Pus could not yet be seen under the skin, but this was already thickened and red over a surface the size of a franc. The inflamed part was washed with alcohol, and dried with blotting paper passed through the flame of an alcohol lamp. A puncture at the thickened portion enabled us to secure a small amount of lymph mixed with blood, which was sowed at the same time as some blood taken from the finger of the hand. The following days, the blood from the finger remained absolutely sterile: but that obtained from the center of the forming furuncle gave an abundant growth of the same small organism as before.

Third observation.—The fourteenth of June, a new furuncle appeared on the neck of the same person. The same examination, the same result, that is to say the development of the microscopic organism previously described and complete sterility of the blood of the general circulation, taken this time at the base of the furuncle outside of the inflamed area.

At the time of making these observations I spoke of them to Dr. Maurice Reynaud, who was good enough to send me a patient who had had furuncles for more than three months. On June thirteenth I made cultures of the pus from a furuncle of this man. The next day there was a general cloudiness of the culture fluids, consisting entirely of the preceding parasite, and of this alone.

Fourth observation.—June fourteenth, the same individual showed me a newly forming furuncle in the left axilla: there was wide-spread thickening and redness of the skin, but no pus was yet apparent. An incision at the center of the thickening showed a small quantity of pus mixed with blood. Sowing, rapid growth for twenty-four hours and the appearance of the same organism. Blood from the arm at a distance from the furuncle remained completely sterile.

June 17, the examination of a fresh furuncle on the same individual gave the same result, the development of a pure culture of the same organism.

Fifth observation.—July twenty-first, Dr. Maurice Reynaud informed me that there was a woman at the Lariboisiere hospital with multiple furuncles. As a matter of fact her back was covered with them, some in active suppuration, others in the ulcerating stage. I took pus from all of these furuncles that had not opened. After a few hours, this pus gave an abundant growth in cultures. The same organism, without admixture, was found. Blood from the inflamed base of the furuncle remained sterile.

In brief, it appears certain that every furuncle contains an aerobic microscopic parasite, to which is due the local inflammation and the pus formation that follows.

Culture fluids containing the minute organism inoculated under the skin of rabbits and guinea-pigs produce abscesses generally small in size and that promptly heal. As long as healing is not complete the pus of the abscesses contains the microscopic organism which produced them. It is therefore living and developing, but its propagation at a distance does not occur. These cultures of which I speak, when injected in small quantities in the jugular vein of guinea pigs show that the minute organism does not grow in the blood. The day after the injection they cannot be recovered even in cultures. I seem to have observed as a general principle, that, provided the blood corpuscles are in good physiological condition it is difficult for aerobic parasites to develop in the blood. I have always thought that this is to be explained by a kind of struggle between the affinity of the blood corpuscles for oxygen and that belonging to the parasite in cultures. Whilst the blood corpuscles carry off, that is, take possession of all the oxygen, the life and development of the parasite become extremely difficult or impossible. It is therefore easily eliminated, digested, if one may use the phrase. I have seen these facts many times in anthrax and chicken-cholera, diseases both of which are due to the presence of an aerobic parasite.

Blood cultures from the general circulation being always sterile in these experiments, it would seem that under the conditions of the furuncular diathesis, the minute parasite does not exist in the blood. That it cannot be cultivated for the reason given, and that it is not abundant is evident; but, from the sterility of the cultures reported (five only) it should not be definitely concluded that the little parasite may not, at some time, be taken up by the blood and transplanted from a furuncle when it is developing to another part of the body, where it may be accidentally lodged, may develop and produce a new furuncle. I am convinced that if, in cases of furuncular diathesis, not merely a few drops but several grams of blood from the general circulation could be placed under cultivation frequent successful growths would be obtained.[1] In the many experiments I have made on the blood in chicken-cholera, I have frequently demonstrated that repeated cultures from droplets of blood do not show an even development even where taken from the same organ, the heart for example, and at the moment when the parasite begins its existence in the blood, which can easily be understood. Once even, it happened that only three out of ten chickens died after inoculation with infectious blood in which the parasite had just began to appear, the remaining seven showed no symptoms whatever. In fact, the microbe, at the moment of beginning its entrance into the blood may exist singly or in minute numbers in one droplet and not at all in its immediate neighbor. I believe therefore that it would be extremely instructive in furunculosis, to find a patient willing to submit to a number of punctures in different parts of the body away from formed or forming furuncles, and thus secure many cultures, simultaneous of otherwise, of the blood of the

[1] This prediction is fully carried out in the present day successful use of considerable amounts of blood in cultures and the resultant frequent demonstrations of bacteria present in the circulation in many infections.— Translator.

general circulation. I am convinced that among them would be found growths of the micro-organism of furuncles.

II. On Osteomyelitis.

Single observation.—I have but one observation relating to this severe disease, and in this Dr. Lannelongue took the initiative. The monograph on osteomyelitis published by this learned practitioner is well known, with his suggestion of the possibility of a cure by trephining the bone and the use of antiseptic washes and dressings. On the fourteenth of February, at the request of Dr. Lannelongue I went to the Sainte-Eugenie hospital, where this skillful surgeon was to operate on a little girl of about twelve years of age. The right knee was much swollen, as well as the whole leg below the calf and a part of the thigh above the knee. There was no external opening. Under chloroform, Dr. Lannelongue made a long incision below the knee which let out a large amount of pus; the tibia was found denuded for a long distance. Three places in the bone were trephined. From each of these, quantities of pus flowed. Pus from inside and outside the bone was collected with all possible precautions and was carefully examined and cultivated later. The direct microscopic study of the pus, both internal and external, was of extreme interest. It was seen that both contained large numbers of the organism similar to that of furuncles, arranged in pairs, in fours and in packets, some with sharp clear contour, others only faintly visible and with very pale outlines. The external pus contained many pus corpuscles, the internal had none at all. It was like a fatty paste of the furuncular organism. Also, it may be noted, that growth of the small organism had begun in less than six hours after the cultures were started. Thus I saw, that it corresponded exactly with the organism of furuncles. The diameter of the individuals was found to be one one-thousandth of a millimeter. If I ventured to express myself so I might say that in this case at least the osteomyelitis was really a furuncle of the bone marrow.[2] It is undoubtedly easy to induce osteomyelitis artificially in living animals.

III. On puerperal fever.

First observation.—On the twelfth of March, 1878, Dr. Hervieux was good enough to admit me to his service in the Maternity to visit a woman delivered some days before and seriously ill with puerperal fever. The lochia were extremely fetid. I found them full of micro-organisms of many kinds. A small amount of blood was obtained from a puncture on the index finger of the left hand, (the finger being first properly washed and dried with a STERILE towel,) and then sowed in chicken bouillon. The culture remained sterile during the following days.

The thirteenth, more blood was taken from a puncture in the finger and this time growth occurred. As death took place on the sixteenth of March at six in the morning, it seems that the blood contained a microscopic parasite at least three days before.

The fifteenth of March, eighteen hours before death, blood from a needle-prick in the left foot was used. This culture also was fertile.

The first culture, of March thirteenth, contained only the organism of furuncles; the next one, that of the fifteenth, contained an organism resembling that of furunculosis, but which always differed enough to make it easy usually to distinguish it. In this way; whilst the parasite of furuncles is arranged in pairs,

[2] This has been demonstrated, as is well known.—Translator.

very rarely in chains of three or four elements, the new one, that of the culture of the fifteenth, occurs in long chains, the number of cells in each being indefinite. The chains are flexible and often appear as little tangled packets like tangled strings of pearls.

The autopsy was performed on the seventeenth at two o'clock. There was a large amount of pus in the peritoneum. It was sowed with all possible precautions. Blood from the basilic and femoral veins was also sowed. So also was pus from the mucous surface of the uterus, from the tubes, and finally that from a lymphatic in the uterine wall. These are the results of these cultures: in all there were the long chains of cells just spoken of above, and nowhere any mixture of other organisms, except in the culture from the peritoneal pus, which, in addition to the long chains, also contained the small pyogenic vibrio which I describe under the name ORGANISM OF PUS in the Note I published with Messrs. Joubert and Chamberland on the thirtieth of April, 1878.[3]

Interpretation of the disease and of the death.—After confinement, the pus that always naturally forms in the injured parts of the uterus instead of remaining pure becomes contaminated with microscopic organisms from outside, notably the organism in long chains and the pyogenic vibrio. These organisms pass into the peritoneal cavity through the tubes or by other channels, and some of them into the blood, probably by the lymphatics. The resorption of the pus, always extremely easy and prompt when it is pure, becomes impossible through the presence of the parasites, whose entrance must be prevented by all possible means from the moment of confinement.

[3] See preceding paper.

Second observation.—The fourteenth of March, a woman died of puerperal fever at the Lariboisiere hospital; the abdomen was distended before death.

Pus was found in abundance by a peritoneal puncture and was sowed; so also was blood from a vein in the arm. The culture of pus yielded the long chains noted in the preceding observation and also the small pyogenic vibrio. The culture from the blood contained only the long chains.

Third observation.—The seventeenth of May, 1879, a woman, three days past confinement, was ill, as well as the child she was nursing. The lochia were full of the pyogenic vibrio and of the organism of furuncles, although there was but a small proportion of the latter. The milk and the lochia were sowed. The milk gave the organism in long chains of granules, and the lochia only the pus organism. The mother died, and there was no autopsy.

On May twenty-eighth, a rabbit was inoculated under the skin of the abdomen with five drops of the preceding culture of the pyogenic vibrio. The days following an enormous abscess formed which opened spontaneously on the fourth of June. An abundantly cheesy pus came from it. About the abscess there was extensive induration. On the eighth of June, the opening of the abscess was larger, the suppuration active. Near its border was another abscess, evidently joined with the first, for upon pressing it with the finger, pus flowed freely from the opening in the first abscess. During the whole of the month of June, the rabbit was sick and the abscesses suppurated, but less and less. In July they closed; the animal was well. There could only be felt some nodules under the skin of the abdomen.

What disturbances might not such an organism carry into the body of a parturient woman, after passing into the peritoneum, the lymphatics or the blood through the maternal placenta! Its presence is much more dangerous than that of the parasite arranged in chains. Furthermore, its development is always threatening, because, as said in the work already quoted (April, 1878) this organism can be easily recovered from many ordinary waters.

I may add that the organism in long chains, and that arranged in pairs are also extremely widespread, and that one of their habitats is the mucous surfaces of the genital tract.[4]

Apparently there is no puerperal parasite, properly speaking. I have not encountered true septicemia in my experiments; but it ought to be among the puerperal affections.

Fourth observation.—On June fourteenth, at the Lariboisiere, a woman was very ill following a recent confinement; she was at the point of death; in fact she did die on the fourteenth at midnight. Some hours before death pus was taken from an abscess on the arm, and blood from a puncture in a finger. Both were sowed. On the next day (the fifteenth) the flask containing the pus from the abscess was filled with long chains of granules. The flask containing the blood was sterile. The autopsy was at ten o'clock on the morning of the sixteenth. Blood from a vein of the arm, pus from the uterine walls and that from a collection in the synovial sac of the knee were all placed in culture media. All showed growth, even the blood, and they all contained the long strings of granules. The peritoneum contained no pus.

[4] When, by the procedure I elsewhere described, urine is removed in a pure condition by the urethra from the bladder, if any chance growth occurs through some error of technic, it is the two organisms of which I have been speaking that are almost exclusively present.

Interpretation of the disease and of the death.—The injury of the uterus during confinement as usual furnished pus, which gave a lodging place for the germs of the long chains of granules. These, probably through the lymphatics, passed to the joints and to some other places, thus being the origin of the metastic abscesses which produced death.

Fifth observation.—On June seventeenth, M. Doleris, a well-known hospital interne, brought to me some blood, removed with the necessary precautions, from a child dead immediately after birth, whose mother, before confinement had had febrile symptoms with chills. This blood, upon cultivation, gave an abundance of the pyogenic vibrio. On the other hand, blood taken from the mother on the morning of the eighteenth (she had died at one o'clock that morning) showed no development whatever, on the nineteenth nor on following days. The autopsy on the mother took place on the nineteenth. It is certainly worthy of note that the uterus, peritoneum and intestines showed nothing special, but the liver was full of metastatic abscesses. At the exit of the hepatic vein from the liver there was pus, and its walls were ulcerated at this place. The pus from the liver abscesses was filled with the pyogenic vibrio. Even the liver tissues, at a distance from the visible abscesses, gave abundant cultures of the same organism.

Interpretation of the disease and of the death.—The pyogenic vibrio, found in the uterus, or which was perhaps already in the body of the mother, since she suffered from chills before confinement, produced metastatic abscesses in the liver and, carried to the blood of the child, there induced one of the forms of infection called purulent, which caused its death.

Sixth observation.—The eighteenth of June, 1879, M. Doleris informed me that a woman confined some days before at the Cochin Hospital, was very ill. On the twentieth of June, blood from a needle-prick in the finger was sowed; the culture was sterile. On July fifteenth, that is to say twenty-five days later, the blood was tried again. Still no growth. There was no organism distinctly recognizable in the lochia: the woman was nevertheless, they told me, dangerously ill and at the point of death. As a matter of fact, she did die on the eighteenth of July at nine in the morning: as may be seen, after a very long illness, for the first observations were made over a month before: the illness was also very painful, for the patient could make no movement without intense suffering.

An autopsy was made on the nineteenth at ten in the morning, and was of great interest. There was purulent pleurisy with a considerable pocket of pus, and purulent false membranes on the walls of the pleura. The liver was bleached, fatty, but of firm consistency, and with no apparent metastatic abscesses. The uterus, of small size, appeared healthy; but on the external surface whitish nodules filled with pus were found. THERE WAS NOTHING IN THE PERITONEUM, WHICH WAS NOT INFLAMED; but there was much pus in the shoulder joints and the symphysis pubis.

The pus from the abscesses, upon cultivation, gave the long chains of granules—not only that of the pleura, but that from the shoulders and a lymphatic of the uterus as well. An interesting thing, but easily understood, was that the blood from a vein in the arm and taken three-quarters of an hour after death was entirely sterile. Nothing grew from the Fallopian tubes nor the broad ligaments.

Interpretation of the disease and of the death.—The pus found in the uterus after confinement became infected with germs of microscopic organisms which grew there, then passed into the uterine lymphatics, and from there went on to produce pus in the pleura and in the articulations.

Seventh observation.—On June eighteenth, M. Doleris informed me that a woman had been confined at the Cochin Hospital five days before and that fears were entertained as to the results of an operation that had been performed, it having been necessary to do an embryotomy. The lochia were sowed on the 18th; there was not the slightest trace of growth the next day nor the day after. Without the least knowledge of this woman since the eighteenth, on the twentieth I ventured to assert that she would get well. I sent to inquire about her. This is the text of the report: "THE WOMAN IS DOING EXTREMELY WELL; SHE GOES OUT TOMORROW"

Interpretation of the facts.—The pus naturally formed on the surface of the injured parts did not become contaminated with organisms brought from without. Natura medicatrix carried it off, that is to say the vitality of the mucous surfaces prevented the development of foreign germs. The pus was easily resorbed, and recovery took place.

I beg the Academy to permit me, in closing, to submit certain definite views, which I am strongly inclined to consider as legitimate conclusions from the facts I have had the honor to communicate to it.

Under the expression PUERPERAL FEVER are grouped very different diseases,[5] but all appearing to be the result of the

[5] Interesting as the starting point of the conception of diseases according to the etiological factor, not by groups of symptoms.—Translator.

growth of common organisms which by their presence infect the pus naturally formed on injured surfaces, which spread by one means or another, by the blood or the lymphatics, to one or another part of the body, and there induce morbid changes varying with the condition of the parts, the nature of the parasite, and the general constitution of the subject.

Whatever this constitution, does it not seem that by taking measures opposing the production of these common parasitic organisms recovery would usually occur, except perhaps when the body contains, before confinement, microscopic organisms, in contaminated internal or external abscesses, as was seen in one striking example (fifth observation). The antiseptic method I believe likely to be sovereign in the vast majority of cases. It seems to me that IMMEDIATELY AFTER CONFINEMENT the application of antiseptics should be begun. Carbolic acid can render great service, but there is another antiseptic, the use of which I am strongly inclined to advise, this is boric acid in concentrated solution, that is, four per cent. at the ordinary temperature. This acid, whose singular influence on cell life has been shown by M. Dumas, is so slightly acid that it is alkaline to certain test papers, as was long ago shown by M. Chevreul, besides this it has no odor like carbolic acid, which odor often disturbs the sick. Lastly, its lack of hurtful effects on mucous membranes, notably of the bladder, has been and is daily demonstrated in the hospitals of Paris. The following is the occasion upon which it was first used. The Academy may remember that I stated before it, and the fact has never been denied, that ammoniacal urine is always produced by a microscopic organism, entirely similar in many respects to the organism of furuncles. Later, in a joint investigation with M. Joubert, we found that a solution of boric acid was easily fatal to these organisms. After that, in 1877,

I induced Dr. Guyon, in charge of the genito-urinary clinic at the Necker hospital, to try injections of a solution of boric acid in affections of the bladder. I am informed by this skilful practitioner that he has done so, and daily observes good results from it. He also tells me that he performs no operation of lithotrity without the use of similar injections. I recall these facts to show that a solution of boric acid is entirely harmless to an extremely delicate mucous membrane, that of the bladder, and that it is possible to fill the bladder with a warm solution of boric acid without even inconvenience.

To return to the confinement cases. Would it not be of great service to place a warm concentrated solution of boric acid, and compresses, at the bedside of each patient; which she could renew frequently after saturating with the solution, and this also after confinement. It would also be acting the part of prudence to place the compresses, before using, in a hot air oven at 150 degrees C., more than enough to kill the germs of the common organisms.[6]

Was I justified in calling this communication "ON THE EXTENSION OF THE GERM THEORY TO THE ETIOLOGY OF CERTAIN COMMON DISEASES?" I have detailed the facts as they have appeared to me and I have mentioned interpretations of them: but I do not conceal from myself that, in medical territory, it is difficult to support one's self wholly on subjective foundations. I do not forget that Medicine and Veterinary practice are foreign to me. I desire judgment and criticism upon all my contributions. Little tolerant of frivolous or prejudiced contradiction, contemptuous of that ignorant criticism which doubts on principle, I welcome with open arms

[6] The adoption of precautions, similar to those here suggested, has resulted in the practically complete disappearance of puerperal fever.—Translator.

the militant attack which has a method in doubting and whose rule of conduct has the motto "More light."

It is a pleasure once more to acknowledge the helpfulness of the aid given me by Messrs. Chamberland and Roux during the studies I have just recorded. I wish also to acknowledge the great assistance of M. Doleris.

ON THE ANTISEPTIC PRINCIPLE OF THE PRACTICE OF SURGERY

Joseph Lister

In the course of an extended investigation into the nature of inflammation, and the healthy and morbid conditions of the blood in relation to it, I arrived several years ago at the conclusion that the essential cause of suppuration in wounds is decomposition brought about by the influence of the atmosphere upon blood or serum retained within them, and, in the case of contused wounds, upon portions of tissue destroyed by the violence of the injury.

To prevent the occurrence of suppuration with all its attendant risks was an object manifestly desirable, but till lately apparently unattainable, since it seemed hopeless to attempt to exclude the oxygen which was universally regarded as the agent by which putrefaction was effected. But when it had been shown by the researches of Pasteur that the septic properties of the atmosphere depended not on the oxygen, or any gaseous constituent, but on minute organisms suspended in it, which owed their energy to their vitality, it occurred to me that decomposition in the injured part might be avoided without excluding the air, by applying as a dressing some material capable of destroying the life of the floating particles. Upon this principle I have based a practice of which I will now attempt to give a short account.

The material which I have employed is carbolic or phenic acid, a volatile organic compound, which appears to exercise a peculiarly destructive influence upon low forms of life, and hence is the most powerful antiseptic with which we are at present acquainted.

The first class of cases to which I applied it was that of compound fractures, in which the effects of decomposition in the injured part were especially striking and pernicious. The results have been such as to establish conclusively the great principle that all local inflammatory mischief and general febrile disturbances which follow severe injuries are due to the irritating and poisonous influence of decomposing blood or sloughs. For these evils are entirely avoided by the antiseptic treatment, so that limbs which would otherwise be unhesitatingly condemned to amputation may be retained, with confidence of the best results.

In conducting the treatment, the first object must be the destruction of any septic germs which may have been introduced into the wounds, either at the moment of the accident or during the time which has since elapsed. This is done by introducing the acid of full strength into all accessible recesses of the wound by means of a piece of rag held in dressing forceps and dipped into the liquid.[1] This I did not venture to do in the earlier cases; but experience has shown that the compound which carbolic acid forms with the blood, and also any portions of tissue killed by its caustic action, including even parts of the bone, are disposed of by absorption and organisation, provided they are afterwards kept from decomposing. We are thus enabled to employ the

[1] The addition of a few drops of water to a considerable quantity of the acid, induces it to assume permanently the liquid form.

antiseptic treatment efficiently at a period after the occurrence of the injury at which it would otherwise probably fail. Thus I have now under my care, in Glasgow Infirmary, a boy who was admitted with compound fracture of the leg as late as eight and one-half hours after the accident, in whom, nevertheless, all local and constitutional disturbance was avoided by means of carbolic acid, and the bones were soundly united five weeks after his admission.

The next object to be kept in view is to guard effectually against the spreading of decomposition into the wound along the stream of blood and serum which oozes out during the first few days after the accident, when the acid originally applied has been washed out or dissipated by absorption and evaporation. This part of the treatment has been greatly improved during the past few weeks. The method which I have hitherto published (see Lancet for Mar. 16th, 23rd, 30th, and April 27th of the present year) consisted in the application of a piece of lint dipped in the acid, overlapping the sound skin to some extent and covered with a tin cap, which was daily raised in order to touch the surface of the lint with the antiseptic. This method certainly succeeded well with wounds of moderate size; and indeed I may say that in all the many cases of this kind which have been so treated by myself or my house-surgeons, not a single failure has occurred. When, however, the wound is very large, the flow of blood and serum is so profuse, especially during the first twenty-four hours, that the antiseptic application cannot prevent the spread of decomposition into the interior unless it overlaps the sound skin for a very considerable distance, and this was inadmissible by the method described above, on account of the extensive sloughing of the surface of the cutis which it would involve. This difficulty has, however, been overcome by employing a paste composed of common whiting (carbonate of lime), mixed with a solution of one part of carbolic acid in four parts of boiled linseed oil so as to form a firm putty. This application contains the acid in too dilute a form to excoriate the skin, which it may be made to cover to any extent that may be thought desirable, while its substance serves as a reservoir of the antiseptic material. So long as any discharge continues, the paste should be changed daily, and, in order to prevent the chance of mischief occurring during the process, a piece of rag dipped in the solution of carbolic acid in oil is put on next the skin, and maintained there permanently, care being taken to avoid raising it along with the putty. This rag is always kept in an antiseptic condition from contact with the paste above it, and destroys any germs which may fall upon it during the short time that should alone be allowed to pass in the changing of the dressing. The putty should be in a layer about a quarter of an inch thick, and may be advantageously applied rolled out between two pieces of thin calico, which maintain it in the form of a continuous sheet, which may be wrapped in a moment round the whole circumference of a limb if this be thought desirable, while the putty is prevented by the calico from sticking to the rag which is next the skin.[2] When all discharge has ceased, the use of the paste is discontinued, but the original rag is left adhering to the skin till healing by scabbing is supposed to be complete. I have at present in the hospital a man with severe compound fracture of both bones of the left leg, caused by direct violence, who, after the cessation of the sanious discharge under the use of the paste, without a drop of

[2] In order to prevent evaporation of the acid, which passes readily through any organic tissue, such as oiled silk or gutta percha, it is well to cover the paste with a sheet of block tin, or tinfoil strengthened with adhesive plaster. The thin sheet lead used for lining tea chests will also answer the purpose, and may be obtained from any wholesale grocer.

pus appearing, has been treated for the last two weeks exactly as if the fracture was a simple one. During this time the rag, adhering by means of a crust of inspissated blood collected beneath it, has continued perfectly dry, and it will be left untouched till the usual period for removing the splints in a simple fracture, when we may fairly expect to find a sound cicatrix beneath it.

We cannot, however, always calculate on so perfect a result as this. More or less pus may appear after the lapse of the first week, and the larger the wound, the more likely this is to happen. And here I would desire earnestly to enforce the necessity of persevering with the antiseptic application in spite of the appearance of suppuration, so long as other symptoms are favorable. The surgeon is extremely apt to suppose that any suppuration is an indication that the antiseptic treatment has failed, and that poulticing or water dressing should be resorted to. But such a course would in many cases sacrifice a limb or a life. I cannot, however, expect my professional brethren to follow my advice blindly in such a matter, and therefore I feel it necessary to place before them, as shortly as I can, some pathological principles intimately connected, not only with the point we are immediately considering, but with the whole subject of this paper.

If a perfectly healthy granulating sore be well washed and covered with a plate of clean metal, such as block tin, fitting its surface pretty accurately, and overlapping the surrounding skin an inch or so in every direction and retained in position by adhesive plaster and a bandage, it will be found, on removing it after twenty-four or forty-eight hours, that little or nothing that can be called pus is present, merely a little transparent fluid, while at the same time there is an entire absence of the unpleasant odour invariably perceived when water dressing is changed. Here the clean metallic surface presents no recesses like those of porous lint for the septic germs to develope in, the fluid exuding from the surface of the granulations has flowed away undecomposed, and the result is the absence of suppuration. This simple experiment illustrates the important fact that granulations have no inherent tendency to form pus, but do so only when subjected to preternatural stimulus. Further, it shows that the mere contact of a foreign body does not of itself stimulate granulations to suppurate; whereas the presence of decomposing organic matter does. These truths are even more strikingly exemplified by the fact that I have elsewhere recorded (Lancet, March 23rd, 1867), that a piece of dead bone free from decomposition may not only fail to induce the granulations around it to suppurate, but may actually be absorbed by them; whereas a bit of dead bone soaked with putrid pus infallibly induces suppuration in its vicinity.

Another instructive experiment is, to dress a granulating sore with some of the putty above described, overlapping the sound skin extensively; when we find, in the course of twenty-four hours, that pus has been produced by the sore, although the application has been perfectly antiseptic; and, indeed, the larger the amount of carbolic acid in the paste, the greater is the quantity of pus formed, provided we avoid such a proportion as would act as a caustic. The carbolic acid, though it prevents decomposition, induces suppuration obviously by acting as a chemical stimulus; and we may safely infer that putrescent organic materials (which we know to be chemically acrid) operate in the same way.

In so far, then, carbolic acid and decomposing substances are alike; viz., that they induce suppuration by chemical stimulation, as distinguished from what may be termed simple inflammatory suppuration, such as that in which ordinary abscesses originate— where the pus appears to be formed in consequence of an excited action of the nerves, independently of any other stimulus. There is, however, this enormous difference between the effects of carbolic acid and those of decomposition; viz., that carbolic acid stimulates only the surface to which it is at first applied, and every drop of discharge that forms weakens the stimulant by diluting it; but decomposition is a self-propagating and self-aggravating poison, and, if it occur at the surface of a severely injured limb, it will spread into all its recesses so far as any extravasated blood or shreds of dead tissue may extend, and lying in those recesses, it will become from hour to hour more acrid, till it requires the energy of a caustic sufficient to destroy the vitality of any tissues naturally weak from inferior vascular supply, or weakened by the injury they sustained in the accident.

Hence it is easy to understand how, when a wound is very large, the crust beneath the rag may prove here and there insufficient to protect the raw surface from the stimulating influence of the carbolic acid in the putty; and the result will be first the conversion of the tissues so acted on into granulations, and subsequently the formation of more or less pus. This, however, will be merely superficial, and will not interfere with the absorption and organisation of extravasated blood or dead tissues in the interior. But, on the other hand, should decomposition set in before the internal parts have become securely consolidated, the most disastrous results may ensue.

I left behind me in Glasgow a boy, thirteen years of age, who, between three and four weeks previously, met with a most severe injury to the left arm, which he got entangled in a machine at a fair. There was a wound six inches long and three inches broad, and the skin was very extensively undermined beyond its limits, while the soft parts were generally so much lacerated that a pair of dressing forceps introduced at the wound and pushed directly inwards appeared beneath the skin at the opposite aspect of the limb. From this wound several tags of muscle were hanging, and among them was one consisting of about three inches of the triceps in almost its entire thickness; while the lower fragment of the bone, which was broken high up, was protruding four inches and a half, stripped of muscle, the skin being tucked in under it. Without the assistance of the antiseptic treatment, I should certainly have thought of nothing else but amputation at the shoulder-joint; but, as the radial pulse could be felt and the fingers had sensation, I did not hesitate to try to save the limb and adopted the plan of treatment above described, wrapping the arm from the shoulder to below the elbow in the antiseptic application, the whole interior of the wound, together with the protruding bone, having previously been freely treated with strong carbolic acid. About the tenth day, the discharge, which up to that time had been only sanious and serous, showed a slight admixture of slimy pus; and this increased till (a few days before I left) it amounted to about three drachms in twenty-four hours. But the boy continued as he had been after the second day, free from unfavorable symptoms, with pulse, tongue, appetite, and sleep natural and strength increasing, while the limb remained as it had been from the first, free from swelling, redness, or pain. I, therefore, persevered with the antiseptic dressing; and, before I left, the discharge was already somewhat less, while the bone was becoming firm. I think it likely that, in that boy's case, I should have found merely a superficial sore had I taken off all the dressings at the end of the three weeks; though, considering the extent of the injury, I thought it prudent to let the month expire before disturbing the rag next the skin. But I feel sure that, if I had resorted to ordinary dressing when the pus first appeared, the progress of the case would have been exceedingly different.

The next class of cases to which I have applied the antiseptic treatment is that of abscesses. Here also the results have been extremely satisfactory, and in beautiful harmony with the pathological principles indicated above. The pyogenic membrane, like the granulations of a sore, which it resembles in nature, forms pus, not from any inherent disposition to do so, but only because it is subjected to some preternatural stimulation. In an ordinary abscess, whether acute or chronic, before it is opened the stimulus which maintains the suppuration is derived from the presence of pus pent up within the cavity. When a free opening is made in the ordinary way, this stimulus is got rid of, but the atmosphere gaining access to the contents, the potent stimulus of decomposition comes into operation, and pus is generated in greater abundance than before. But when the evacuation is effected on the antiseptic principle, the pyogenic membrane, freed from the influence of the former stimulus without the substitution of a new one, ceases to suppurate (like the granulations of a sore under metallic dressing), furnishing merely a trifling amount of clear serum, and, whether the opening be dependent or not, rapidly contracts and coalesces. At the same time any constitutional symptoms previously occasioned by the accumulation of the matter are got rid of without the slightest risk of the irritative fever or hectic hitherto so justly dreaded in dealing with large abscesses.

In order that the treatment may be satisfactory, the abscess must be seen before it is opened. Then, except in very rare and peculiar cases,[3] there are no septic organisms in the contents, so that it is needless to introduce carbolic acid into the interior. Indeed, such a procedure would be objectionable, as it would stimulate the pyogenic membrane to unnecessary suppuration. All that is requisite is to guard against the introduction of living atmospheric germs from without, at the same time that free opportunity is afforded for the escape of the discharge from within.

I have so lately given elsewhere a detailed account of the method by which this is effected (Lancet, July 27th, 1867), that I shall not enter into it at present further than to say that the means employed are the same as those described above for the super-ficial dressing of compound fractures; viz., a piece of rag dipped into the solution of carbolic acid in oil to serve as an antiseptic curtain, under cover of which the abscess is evacuated by free incision, and the antiseptic paste to guard against decomposition occurring in the stream of pus that flows out beneath it; the dressing being changed daily until the sinus is closed.

The most remarkable results of this practice in a pathological point of view have been afforded by cases where the formation of pus depended on disease of bone. Here the abscesses, instead of forming exceptions to the general class in the obstinacy of the suppuration, have resembled the rest in yielding in a few days only a trifling discharge, and frequently the production of pus has ceased from the moment of the evacuation of the original

[3] As an instance of one of these exceptional cases, I may mention that of an abscess in the vicinity of the colon, and afterwards proved by post-mortem examination to have once communicated with it. Here the pus was extremely offensive when evacuated, and exhibited vibrios under the microscope.

contents. Hence it appears that caries, when no longer labouring as heretofore under the irritation of decomposing matter, ceases to be an opprobrium of surgery, and recovers like other inflammatory affections. In the publication before alluded to, I have mentioned the case of a middle-aged man with a psoas abscess depending in diseased bone, in whom the sinus finally closed after months of patient perseverance with the antiseptic treatment. Since that article was written I have had another instance of abscess equally gratifying, but the differing in the circumstance that the disease and the recovery were more rapid in their course. The patient was a blacksmith, who had suffered four and a half months before I saw him from symptoms of ulceration of cartilage in the left elbow. These had latterly increased in severity so as to deprive him entirely of his night's rest and of appetite. I found the region of the elbow greatly swollen, and on careful examination found a fluctuating point at the outer aspect of the articulation. I opened it on the antiseptic principle, the incision evidently penetrating to the joint, giving exit to a few drachms of pus. The medical gentleman under whose care he was (Dr. Macgregor, of Glasgow) supervised the daily dressing with the carbolic acid paste till the patient went to spend two or three weeks at the coast, when his wife was entrusted with it. Just two months after I opened the abscess, he called to show me the limb, stating that the discharge had been, for at least two weeks, as little as it was then, a trifling moisture upon the paste, such as might be accounted for by the little sore caused by the incision. On applying a probe guarded with an antiseptic rag, I found that the sinus was soundly closed, while the limb was free from swelling or tenderness; and, although he had not attempted to exercise it much, the joint could already be moved through a considerable angle. Here the antiseptic principle had effected the restoration of a joint, which, on any other known system of treatment, must have been excised.

Ordinary contused wounds are, of course, amenable to the same treatment as compound fractures, which are a complicated variety of them. I will content myself with mentioning a single instance of this class of cases. In April last, a volunteer was discharging a rifle when it burst, and blew back the thumb with its metacarpal bone, so that it could be bent back as on a hinge at the trapezial joint, which had evidently been opened, while all the soft parts between the metacarpal bones of the thumb and forefinger were torn through. I need not insist before my present audience on the ugly character of such an injury. My house-surgeon, Mr. Hector Cameron, applied carbolic acid to the whole raw surface, and completed the dressing as if for compound fracture. The hand remained free from pain, redness or swelling, and with the exception of a shallow groove, all the wound consolidated without a drop of matter, so that if it had been a clean cut, it would have been regarded as a good example of primary union. The small granulating surface soon healed, and at present a linear cicatrix alone tells of the injury he has sustained, while his thumb has all its movements and his hand a fine grasp.

If the severest forms of contused and lacerated wounds heal thus kindly under the antiseptic treatment, it is obvious that its application to simple incised wounds must be merely a matter of detail. I have devoted a good deal of attention to this class, but I have not as yet pleased myself altogether with any of the methods I have employed. I am, however, prepared to go so far as to say that a solution of carbolic acid in twenty parts of water, while a mild and cleanly application, may be relied on for destroying any septic germs that may fall upon the wound during the performance of an operation; and also that, for preventing the subsequent introduction of others, the paste above described, applied as for compound fractures, gives excellent results. Thus I have had a case of strangulated inguinal hernia in which it was necessary to take away half a pound of thickened omentum, heal without any deep-seated suppuration or any tenderness of the sac or any fever; and amputations, including one immediately below the knee, have remained absolutely free from constitutional symptoms.

Further, I have found that when the antiseptic treatment is efficiently conducted, ligatures may be safely cut short and left to be disposed of by absorption or otherwise. Should this particular branch of the subject yield all that it promises, should it turn out on further trial that when the knot is applied on the antiseptic principle, we may calculate as securely as if it were absent on the occurrence of healing without any deep-seated suppuration, the deligation of main arteries in their continuity will be deprived of the two dangers that now attend it, viz., those of secondary haemorrhage and an unhealthy state of the wound. Further, it seems not unlikely that the present objection to tying an artery in the immediate vicinity of a large branch may be done away with; and that even the innominate, which has lately been the subject of an ingenious experiment by one of the Dublin surgeons, on account of its well-known fatality under the ligature for secondary haemorrhage, may cease to have this unhappy character when the tissues in the vicinity of the thread, instead of becoming softened through the influence of an irritating decomposing substance, are left at liberty to consolidate firmly near an unoffending though foreign body.

It would carry me far beyond the limited time which, by the rules of the Association, is alone at my disposal, were I to enter into the various applications of the antiseptic principle in the several special departments of surgery.

There is, however, one point more that I cannot but advert to, viz., the influence of this mode of treatment upon the general healthiness of an hospital. Previously to its introduction the two large wards in which most of my cases of accident and of operation are treated were among the unhealthiest in the whole surgical division of the Glasgow Royal Infirmary, in consequence apparently of those wards being unfavorably placed with reference to the supply of fresh air; and I have felt ashamed when recording the results of my practice, to have so often to allude to hospital gangrene or pyaemia. It was interesting, though melancholy, to observe that whenever all or nearly all the beds contained cases with open sores, these grievous complications were pretty sure to show themselves; so that I came to welcome simple fractures, though in themselves of little interest either for myself or the students, because their presence diminished the proportion of open sores among the patients. But since the antiseptic treatment has been brought into full operation, and wounds and abscesses no longer poison the atmosphere with putrid exhalations, my wards, though in other respects under precisely the same circumstances as before, have completely changed their character; so that during the last nine months not a single instance of pyaemia, hospital gangrene, or erysipelas has occurred in them.

As there appears to be no doubt regarding the cause of this change, the importance of the fact can hardly be exaggerated.

A METHOD OF ANTISEPTIC TREATMENT APPLICABLE TO WOUNDED SOLDIERS IN THE PRESENT WAR

HAVING been requested to furnish some rules for the antiseptic treatment of wounded soldiers in the present war, I venture to suggest the following plan, in the hope that it will combine efficiency with the simplicity and facility of execution essential under such circumstances.

Wash the wound thoroughly, and also the surrounding skin, with a saturated solution of crystallised carbolic (phenic) acid in water, one part of the acid to twenty of water, introducing the fluid by means of a syringe, and manipulating the parts freely so as to cause the lotion to penetrate into all the interstices of the wound; and at the same time squeeze out such clots of blood as it may contain. The fluid should be introduced repeatedly to insure its thorough penetration. Tie any bleeding vessels with properly prepared antiseptic catgut, cutting off the ends of the thread near the knot. If the surgeon do not possess this article, the arteries should, if possible, be secured by torsion; but for the sake of cases in which a ligature would be absolutely indispensable, some silk or linen thread should be kept steeping in a strong oily solution of carbolic acid, or, if very fine silk be used, it may be rendered antiseptic by steeping for a few minutes in the watery solution. When silk or linlen is employed, the ends of the ligatures should be left projecting at the wound. While the antiseptic lotion is in the wound, extract if possible any foreign material that may have been introduced, such as a bullet or a portion of the patient's clothes; and if any specula of bone exist entirely detached from the soft parts, remove such as can be readily reached, disregarding those which are of very small size orinconvenient of access. Then place upon the wound two or three layers of oiled silk smeared on both sides with a solution of carbolic acid in five parts of any of the fixed oils-olive, almcnd, linseed, etc.-the oiled silk being made large enough to cover the raw surface completely and slightly overlap the surrounding skin. Next apply, without loss of time, lint, charpie, or cloth (linen or cotton), well steeped in the oily solution of the acid, the cloth or lint being folded sufficiently to produce a layer at least a quarter of an inch in thickness, and extending a considerable distance, say three inches, beyond the oiled silk in all directions, the outer layer being made somewhat larger than the rest, so that the margin of the mass of cloth may be thin. Cover the oily cloth with a piece of thin gutta-percha tissue sufficiently large to overlap it on all sides by an inch or more, and retain it securely in position by a roller steeped in the antiseptic oil. Round this again wrap a still larger piece of folded cloth, say a folded towel, also steeped in the oily solution of carbolic acid, and cover it with a piece of oiled Silk or gutta-percha.

With a view to the intelligent application of this dressing, it will be well to state briefly its rationale. The watery solution is applied in order to destroy once for all any septic particles that may have been introduced into the wound; and the oily solution is employed to prevent the spread of putrefactive fermentation into the wound from without. The oiled silk, which is but slightly permeable to carbolic acid, protects the raw surface from the irritation of the acid in the oily cloth, and permits it to heal as under a scab. But though the ultimate office of the oiled silk is to protect the wound from the irritation of the antiseptic, it must itself be antiseptic at the time of application, and is therefore smeared with the oil, which in the course of no long time loses its carbolic acid by diffusion into the wound beneath. The substantial and widely extending oily cloth serves as a store of the antiseptic; but the bloody and serous discharge soaking into the porous cloth tends to wash away the oil and deprive the dressing of its antiseptic character; hence the necessity for the gutta-percha, which prevents the discharge from making its way directly outwards from the wound, and so establishing a road for the penetration of putrefaction inwards. At the same time the gutta-percha, though impermeable to watery or oily fluid, being readily permeated by carbolic acid, permits the antiseptic ingredient to pass in through it from the outer cloth and act upon the discharge that flows out beneath the overlapping margins of the gutta-percha. The outer cloth is intended to be changed as occasion may require, in order to keep up the supply of the antiseptic, while the gutta-percha and all beneath it constitute a more permanent application. The layer of gutta-percha or oiled silk outside the external cloth is to prevent the oil in that cloth from being wasted by soaking out into the surrounding articles of clothing, etc.; or, still worse, neutralised chemically by the penetration inwards of putrid blood or other discharges from the ambulance waggon or bedding. The circumferential part of the deeper cloth will, in consequence of its thinness, be kept completely antiseptic by the carbolic acid which passes inwards through the gutta-percha, while the deeper layers of the thicker portion over the wound will probably in a few days be destitute of antiseptic, and therefore of stimulating, properties; hence the oiled silk, though desirable in order to insure the absence of "antiseptic suppuration!", is by no means an essential part of the treatment, and if none of it be at hand the procedure may in other respects be conducted in the same way without it. Again, if the surgeon have no gutta-percha at his disposal, the risk that would otherwise arise from the permeability of the dressing may be overcome by frequently changing an external antiseptic cloth, or by treating its surface every few hours with the antiseptic oil.

The changing of the outer cloth will require care in order to avoid raising the edge of the gutta-percha along with it, and so admitting septic air towards the wound. It may be done with perfect security by having the cloth consist of two parts, one covering each half of the gutta-percha, and, as one half is raised, throwing a stream of watery solution (I to 40) with a syringe upon the margin of the gutta-percha, a fresh oiled cloth being at once applied before the other portion of the former cloth is removed. If sufficient time cannot be spared for changing the outer cloth in this careful manner, it will be better for the surgeon to content himself with pouring fresh oily solution upon the exterior of the cloth without disturbing it, taking care that the oil enter well beneath its margins. I would advise that this should be done in preference where a large number of wounded have to be treated by one surgeon.

The strong oily solution (I to 5) would irritate the skin if used continuously: after the first dressing a solution of half the strength should be employed, and after a few days it may be reduced to I to 20 if excoriation should occur.

The times of changing the outer cloth, or treating it with fresh oil, should be in accordance with the amount of discharge. During the first twenty-four hours the effusion of blood and serum is necessarily profuse, and it will be well that fresh oil be applied to the outer cloth within twelve hours of the first dressing, or even in six hours if there should be unusual oozing. On the second day, also, in the case of a large wound, two dressings in the twenty-four hours will be desirable. After this, if all go well, the discharge will diminish quickly, and a daily renewal of the antiseptic supply will be sufficient; and when five or six days have passed, to apply the oil once in two days will be all that will be required. This, however, should be continued after discharge has ceased entirely, till sufficient time has passed to insure that the wound has healed by scabbing, or at least has been converted into a superficial sore.

The earlier the case comes under treatment the greater will be the prospect of success, but even after the lapse of thirty-six hours it need not be altogether despaired of. In the case of compound fractures, the essential objects of the treatment may be attained by using splints constructed of stout iron wire bent into the form of the margin of a lateral splint, and strengthened by cross pieces here and there. Such splints can be readily extemporized by the surgeon himself, by help of two pairs of wire-forceps. The splints should be applied one at each side of the limb, without any padding opposite the seat of injury except the dressing above described, but padded elsewhere with any suitable soft material, an interval being left between such padding and the dressing. The outer layer of oiled silk or gutta-percha should be applied outside the splints, so that all that will be requisite in order to apply oil to the outer cloth will be to take off the oiled silk with its retaining bandage, and pour on the oil through the ample intervals between the wires. Or the splints might be applied immediately external to the bandage that retains the deeper layer of gutta percha, leaving the outer cloth to be wrapped round external to the splints, cotton or charpie imbued with the antiseptic oil being tucked in under the splints to keep the margins of the gutta-percha in apposition with the limb, the cotton being changed as often as the cloth itself.

For the sake of the general healthiness of the atmosphere of the crowded military hospitals, it is extremely desirable that even superficial granulating sores should be treated antiseptically. This may be done consistently with rapid healing by washing the sore with watery solution of carbolic acid (one to twenty), and covering it with two or three layers of oiled sick smeared with the oily solution (one to twenty), with well overlapping folded cloth steeped in similar oil, and over all a piece of gutta-percha tissue and bandage.

I have suggested in the above method the employment of such materials as are likely to be accessible to the surgeons of both armies. Other means exist, in some respects very superior. But the supply of these is, at present limited, and those who possess them probably understand their use.

ON THE EARLY
STAGES OF
INFLAMMATION

Joseph Lister

INTRODUCTION

THE morbid process designated by the term Inflammation, being one to which every organ and probably every tissue of the body is liable, and comprehending as it does in its progress and consequences by far the greater number of the ills to which flesh is heir, possesses a deeper interest for the physician or surgeon than any other material subject which could be named. The practical importance of inquiries tending to elucidate the essential nature of this process, has been for centuries recognized by all enlightened members of the medical profession; for it is obvious that just views regarding it must tend to promote the establishment of sound principles in the treatment of the diseases which it produces. At the present day more especially, when theory is allowed such free scope, and is permitted to attack the most time-honoured rules of practice, we stand in peculiar need of the beacon-light of correct pathology to enable us to steer a safe course amid the various conflicting opinions which assail us. Yet so far from our knowledge of inflammation being in a satisfactory condition, authorities are at variance upon the fundamental question, whether it is to be regarded, in accordance with JOHN HUNTER'S opinion, as active in its nature, and consisting in an exaltation of the functions of the affected part, or whether it should not rather be considered a passive result of diminished functional activity.

In seeking for the solution of this great problem, we cannot expect to gain much from the contemplation of the more advanced stages and results of inflammation, such as copious exudation of lymph, suppuration, ulceration, or gangrene. When any one of these has taken place, the nature of the original disease is masked to a great extent by the subsequent changes; and the cell-development which occurs in lymph after its effusion, is no more proof of activity in the inflammatory process, than the loss of the vital powers in gangrene can be accepted as evidence in the opposite direction. It is upon the first deviations from health that the essential character of the morbid state will be most unequivocally stamped, and it is therefore to the early stages of inflammation that attention must be chiefly directed in this inquiry.

If the palm of the hand be chafed by long-continued friction, as for example in rowing a boat, the first thing that will be observed, when attention has been directed to the part by a feeling of uneasiness, will be that the skin is redder than natural, implying that the vessels are abnormally loaded with blood, and if the irritation be continued, the cuticle will be raised in the form of a blister. If, now, the loosened epidermis be artificially removed on the earliest occurrence of effusion, a scarlet raw surface will be exposed; and on pressing the tender dermis firmly with the finger, and suddenly removing the pressure, it will be found that while the redness will for the most part have momentarily disappeared, there will be many minute red points from which the blood cannot be expelled. This shows that, while the blood is in part still free to move, there are some minute vessels completely clogged with it. Again, if a portion of mustard be placed on the skin covering the dorsal aspect of one of the fingers, abnormal redness will very speedily be produced, which in the first instance disappears completely on pressure; but, if the mustard has been kept on long enough, can be only imperfectly dispelled; and if the application be still longer continued, vesication will be the result. I had lately the opportunity of examining the brain of a man who had died of tetanus, complicated with incipient meningitis; the post mortem appearance of the latter being maculiform congestion of the pia mater. Having stripped off a portion of the affected membrane, and carefully washed away with a camel's-hair brush the cerebral substance adhering to it, I applied the microscope to one of the affected spots, and found that all the minute vessels were filled with crimson blood, while those of the surrounding parts were comparatively pale. It was evident that the red corpuscles were, in the former, so closely crammed together as to produce the appearance of a uniform mass, while in the latter they were present only in their usual proportion to the liquor sanguinis. Thus it appears that in the human subject, inflammation, whether induced by mechanical irritation or by an acrid application such as mustard, or of spontaneous origin, is characterized at an early period by a certain amount of obstruction to the progress of the blood through the minute vessels; a phenomenon, which it is therefore of great importance to understand.

It fortunately happens, that we have, in the transparent web of the frog's foot, an opportunity of observing with the utmost facility the circulation of the blood in the living animal, and of watching the effects produced upon it by irritating causes. It may naturally appear very doubtful whether observations made upon creatures so low in the animal kingdom as the Amphibia, can with propriety be brought to bear upon human pathology. A few facts will, however, suffice to show that no such doubts need be entertained.

If a portion of moistened mustard be placed upon the web of a frog, tied out under the microscope, the blood-vessels will soon be found abnormally red; and if the application be continued long enough, all the capillaries will become choked with corpuscles so closely packed as to present the appearance of a uniform crimson mass; and by and by the epidermis will be found raised in the form of a blister over the part on which the mustard lay. These effects are precisely similar to those which we have seen to be produced by it upon the human skin; and before effusion has taken place, the vessels of the affected part exactly resemble those of the congested spot of inflamed pia mater above described. Again, if dry heat be made to act upon a part of the frog's foot, there will result, in proportion to the elevation of the temperature and the duration of its action, undue redness of the vessels from accumulation of the blood-corpuscles; and if the burn have been sufficiently severe, vesication will soon take place as in the human subject. These and other similar cases indicate that the early stages of inflammation are alike in man and in the frog, and this conclusion is fully confirmed by examination of the bat's wing, which furnishes the means of watching the effects of irritants upon mammalian circulation. The very small size of the blood-corpuscles, and some other circumstances, render that animal much less suitable for the investigation than the frog; but with the use of high powers of the microscope and a little pains, the same sort of experiments can be made with both: and the careful observations of Messrs. PAGET and WHARTON JONES, and, I may add, also my own more limited experience with the bat, have shown that in all the details that can be observed, a complete similarity obtains between the effects of irritation upon the circulation in the two creatures. We may therefore rest fully satisfied that conclusions arrived at from the study of the early stages of inflammation in the foot of the frog will apply in all strictness to the same morbid process in man.

It is well known that the field of observation thus afforded has not been allowed to remain uncultivated. Since the microscope has been brought to its present state of perfection, not to speak of a previous period, men of established scientific reputation have devoted much patient labour to it; and any one who now enters upon this inquiry has the great advantage of possessing faithful records of accurate observations made by many able predecessors. But the number and discordance of the views entertained by different authorities regarding the cause of the "stasis" of the blood in inflammation, are sufficient evidence either that the subject demands further investigation, or else that it lies beyond the reach of human means of research.

Having been called upon in the capacity of a teacher of surgery to attempt an explanation of the matter to others, I felt bound to do my best, by personal observation, to form a judgement for myself; and several new facts which I have unexpectedly met with appear to throw such fresh and clear light upon the nature of disease, that I venture to submit them to the Royal Society.

SECTION I. *On the Aggregation of the Corpuscles of the Blood.*

The tendency of the corpuscles of the blood to aggregate together, constitutes, as we shall see, an important element in the cause of the obstruction which they experience in the vessels of an inflamed part. It is therefore desirable that we should be acquainted with the nature of the phenomenon.

If a drop of human blood just shed is placed between two plates of glass and examined with the microscope, the red corpuscles are seen to become applied to one another by their flat surfaces, so as to form long cylindrical masses like piles of money, as first observed in 1827 by my father and Dr. HODGKIN and the terminal corpuscles of each "rouleau" adhering to other rouleaux, a network is produced with intervals of colourless liquor sanguinis. Rapid movement of the blood prevents this occurrence, but it commences as soon as the corpuscles approach to a state of quiescence, and I have seen short rouleaux already present in a drop drawn from my own finger within ten seconds of its emission. In this respect the aggregation of the red corpuscles differs from the coagulation of the fibrine, which does not begin till some minutes after withdrawal from the vessels. There is, in fact, no connexion whatever between the two processes, as is clear from the circumstance that if a drop of blood is stirred with a needle while coagulation is taking place, so as to remove the whole of the fibrine, the corpuscles, which have been separated from one another by the agitation to which they have been subjected, aggregate again in the serum in the same manner as they did at first in the liquor sanguinis. The beautifully regular form of the long masses of corpuscles has suggested to some persons the idea of the operation of some peculiar vital attraction in their formation, while by others the aggregation has been supposed due to merely physical causes, but has never, I think, received a complete explanation. For my own part, I am satisfied that the rouleaux are simply the result of the biconcave form of the red discs, together with a certain, though not very great degree of adhesiveness, which retains them pretty firmly attached together when in the position most favourable for its operation, namely, when the margins of their concave surfaces are applied accurately together, but allows them to slip upon one another when in any other position. There is never to be seen anything indicating the existence of an attractive force drawing the corpuscles towards each other: they merely stick together when brought into contact by accidental causes. Their adhesiveness does not afflict tllemselves alone, but other substances also, as may be seen when blood is in motion in an extremely thin film between two plates of glass, when they may be observed sticking for a longer or shorter time to one of the surfaces of the glass, each one dragging behind it a short tail-like process; and as the movement of the blood diminishes so as to permit the formation of rouleaux, the latter may be not unfrequently seen adhering in the same way by one of their terminal corpuscles.

That the cylindrical character of the aggregated masses is an accidental result of the shape of the blood-discs, is evident from the fact, that in the frog, although the same tendency to agglutination of he corpuscles exists as in Mammalia, yet, as their bi-convex form renders it mechanically impossible for them o be applied to one another throughout their entire circumference, hey become arranged in groups of an irregular form, as is shown in the annexed sketcli of blood contained in a small vein of the frog's web.

Again, different specimens of mammalian blood differ very much in the amount of adhesiveness of their corpuscles; and when this property exists beyond a certain degree, the cliscs stick together by any parts that happen to come first in contact, and retain that position more or less, so that the result is the formation, not of rouleaux, but of irregular confused masses. The most striking example which I have seen of this was presented by the blood of a bat, which had lived some days after having been severely wounded. In that case, chains of red discs might be seen adhering firmly by their edges, notwithstanding considerable force of traction operating upon them, and before they at last gave way, tail-like processes of considerable length.were drawn out between every pair of corpuscles, indicating that they were very adhesive. These facts seem sufficient proof of the correctness of the view above expressed regarding the cause of the rouleaux.

The adhesiveness of the red corpuscles does not appear to be a vital property. When the fibrine has been removed from a drop of blood during the progress of coagulation, the rouleaux will form again, after being broken up, as many times as the experiment is repeated, until the blood becomes thick from dryness; and if evaporation be prevented by Canada balsam placed round the plate of thin glass, with suitable precaution against the approximation of the two plates, the rouleaux will remain perfect for several days (e. g. fourteen in one experiment of the kind), after which the very slow chemical action of the balsam upon the blood gradually renders it confusedly red and opaque. Gum mixed with blood seems to preserve it, like a pickle, from decomposition for a very considerable period; and if a piece of met lint be suspended above such a specimen so as to prevent evaporation, the corpuscles will retain their adhesiveness for a long time (e. g. twenty-four days in one instance), until the water communicated to the mixture by the artificially damp atmosphere gradually renders them non-adhesive. These experiments were made in winter, when the low temperature preveilts rapid decomposition; but it appears unlikely that even at that period of the year a part of the human body should retain any vital properties after having been left three and a half weeks mixed with strong gum, which, it is to be observed, alters very much the form and appearance of the corpuscles.

Both in man and in the frog the white corpuscles also are found aggregated together more or less in a drop of blood examined microscopically, and indeed they adhere much more closely than the red ones both to the glass and to one another; but as they are not disc-shaped, but globular, they do not become grouped into rouleaux, but into irregular masses, which, in consequence of their colourless and transparent character, are apt to pass unnoticed, or to be mistaken for masses of coagulated fibrine. If a portion of blood be allowed to run in between two plates of glass nearly in contact with one another, the white corpuscles will be found sticking together near the edge of the glass at which the blood entered, the blood having been as it were filtered of white corpuscles as it passed on; and this is not due to the greater size of the colourless corpuscles than the red, for I have seen it occur with frog's blood when there was room enough between the plates for the red corpuscles to lie edgewise, their transverse dimensions being greater than the diameter of a white corpuscle.

The red corpuscles also often adhere to the colourless ones.

It will be seen hereafter that the corpuscles of blood within the vessels of the king body present great varieties of adhesiveness, according to the amount of irritation to which a part may be subjected; such variations are also met with in blood outside the body, in consequence of differences in the quality of the plasma.

If a drop of very thick solution of gum-arabic, freshly prepared and free from acidity, be added to about four drops of blood, the red corpuscles of the mixture will be found to aggregate much more speedily and more closely than those of ordinary blood, a fact ascertained some years ago by Mr. WHARTON JONES and some other observers. The result is the formation of dense orange masses with large colourless interspaces, but without much regular appearance of rouleaux. On closely examining such a specimen, the red discs are seen to be much diminished in breadth and increased in thickness, and exhibit an extreme degree of adhesiveness, sticking together indifferently by their edges, or any other parts that happen to come first; and if one of the masses be stretched so as to break, the separating corpuscles become drawn out into long viscid processes, which at length give way in the middle, and each half is drawn into its respective corpuscle.

This remarkable effect cannot be accounted for by the mere viscidity of the plasma, which would not make the corpuscles adhere to each other more intimately than usual, unless they had themselves experienced some change, of which, indeed, their altered form is conclusive evidence. Further, if a very small quantity of acetic acid be added to the gum before mixing it with the blood, the corpuscles will be found to have lost altogether their adhesive character, although the mixture may be made viscid to any degree that may be desired. A little acid perspiration on the finger appears to prevent entirely the formation of rouleaux in a drop of blood taken from it; but after the finger has been washed, the usual appearances present themselves when more blood is drawn. Diminished adhesiveness of the red corpuscles is also the earliest evidence of the chemical action of tincture of cantharides and croton oil on the blood of the frog. A similar effect is produced when a drop of human blood is shed into a little fresh almond or olive oil on a plate of glass, and stirred slightly so as to break up the blood into minute drops. On microscopic examination of such a mixture, one sees the red discs aggregated as usual in the interior of the larger drops; but at their exterior, which is in contact with the oil, and throughout the smaller drops, the corpuscles are somewhat altered in form, being of less diameter, but thicker, though still in the form of discs, and at the same time they are found to have lost every trace of a tendency to adhere together; and when present in a thin layer of blood they stand apart at equal distances from one another, as if exercising a mutual repulsion, at the same time exhibiting molecular movements. If a drop of blood freshly shed upon a glass plate be stirred with a needle in an atmosphere of chloroform vapour, the rouleaux will be found to form less perfectly in proportion to the time that the chloroform has acted, until, if the period be as long as thirty seconds, the corpuscles will be all cup-shaped, and will exhibit no disposition to aggregate. But no effect is produced on the formation of the rouleaux by stirring a drop of blood in the same way for a much longer time in an atmosphere free from chloroform. The aggregation of the corpuscles is not prevented merely by their becoming cup-shaped, and therefore unable to apply themselves to each other as usual. For the vapour of caustic ammonia, while it renders the corpuscles cup-shaped, seems rather to increase than to diminish their adhesiveness and aggregating tendency, and a temperature of about 32 degrees Fahrenheit as similar effects with the alkali. Even in the mixture of blood and gum many of the corpuscles are cup-shaped, though adhering together with peculiar tenacity.

Whether or not it will ever be possible to explain these curious facts upon chemical principles seems very doubtful; but in the meantime, what appears most striking about them, and what most concerns the present inquiry, is that great effects may be produced upon the adhesiveness of the red corpuscles, both in the way of increase and diminution, by very slight changes in the chemical qualities of the plasma.

The galvanic current produces no effect upon the aggregation of the red corpuscles, either of man or of the frog, as I have ascertained by placing the fine platinum wire extremities of the poles of a powerful battery a short distance from one another between two slips of glass beneath the microscope, then completing the circuit by shedding a drop of blood between the plates, and immediately observing the result. In several such experiments I invariably found that aggregation took place as usual, and the only effect produced by the galvanism was a chemical change in the blood, dependent on electrolysis, gradually developing itself in the immediate vicinity of the poles, and causing solution of the corpuscles.

The buffy coat in inflammatory blood was first explained by Mr. WHARTON JONES, who showed that it resulted from the red corpuscles aggregating more closely than usual, and therefore falling more rapidly through the lighter plasma, so as to leave the upper portions completely before the occurrence of coagulation. It was supposed by the same authority that this peculiarity of the red discs was due to increased fibrine in solution, rendering the liquor sanguinis abnormally viscid, and so operating like the admixture of gum above alluded to. But the fact that the corpuscles aggregate as closely after the fibrine has been removed as before, appears quite opposed to such a view. I have examined many drops of my own blood, before and after the removal of its fibrine, with the special object of ascertaining this point, and have never been able to detect any material difference between the aggregation in the two sets of cases. In the blood of the bat before mentioned, which was probably suffering constitutionally from inflammation, the corpuscles continued to retain their excessive adhesiveness for a whole hour after coagulation of the fibrine. I once made a similar observation on a specimen of horse's blood, which, as is well known, presents the buffy coat in the state of health. Having divided the clot vertically several hours after coagulation had occurred, my attention was attracted, on looking at the section, by minute red points, like grains of sand, lying in the lower part of the buff, just above the coloured portion of the coagulum. On microscopic examination of a small piece containing some of them, they proved, as I expected, to be masses of aggregated red corpuscles, but with the peculiarity of being compact and globular instead of presenting the usual appearance of a network of rouleaux, and it was evident that the corpuscles had been excessively adhesive at the time when aggregation took place. Some of the red discs were now squeezed out from the fibrinous mass in which they lay, and as they escaped into the surrounding serum they at once adhered firmly in that fluid, forming again compact globular masses, such as, if in freshly-drawn blood, would necessarily give rise to the buffy coat; so that their adhesiveness seemed to have been in no way affected by the withdrawal of the fibrine from solution. It may of course be urged, that the fibrine, when in solution, may have impressed upon the corpuscles an adhesiveness which they retained after soaking for hours in serum, but this seems a very unlikely hypothesis. I suspect, therefore, that the peculiarities of the corpuscles of inflammatory blood are the result of other changes than the excess of fibrine.

From the facts detailed in this section, it appears that the aggregation of the corpuscles of blood removed from the body depends on their possessing a certain degree of mutual adhesiveness, which is much greater in the colourless globules than in the red discs; and that, in the latter, this property, though apparently not depending upon vitality, is capable of remarkable variations in consequence of very slight chemical changes in the liquor sanguinis.

SECTION II: *On the Structure and Functions of the Bloodvessels.*

An acquaintance with the anatomy and physiology of the vascular system is indispensable to a successful study of the deviations from health exhibited in the circulation of the blood through the vessels of an inflamed part; it is not, however, intended to give here a full account of the subject, but merely to dwell upon some important points on which differences of opinion prevail.

It has long been a debated question whether or not the capillaries possess contractility, and there is still some difference of opinion among authorities upon the subject. with a view to throwing light upon this important point, I investigated carefully the structure of the minute vessels of the frog's foot; dissecting them out from between the layers of skin composing the web, so as to render their constituent material capable of clear definition with the microscope. The chief results have been communicated to the Royal Society of Edinburgh, in a paper that will shortly appear in their Transactions, "On the Structure of Involuntary Muscular Fiber." I need therefore merely repeat here, that while the capillaries were proved to consist, as has been long known, merely of a delicate homogeneous membrane beset with occasional nuclei, the minute arteries, some of them even less in calibre than average capillaries, were found to possess three distinct coats, namely, an external layer of cellular tissue, in variable quantity, longitudinally arranged, an internal extremely delicate lining membrane, and an intermediate circular coat, which constituted the principal bulk of the vascular parietes, and which, when highly magnified, was found to consist of a single layer of muscular fibre-cells, each wound spirally round the internal membrane so as to encircle it from one and a half to two and a half times.

Now when we consider the properties of muscular fibre-cells, which, as is shown in the paper referred to, are capable of contracting in the pig's intestine as much as to one-tenth of their length, it is impossible to conceive a more efficient mechanism for the constriction of a tube than is provided in these minute arteries. On the other hand, the capillaries are totally destitute of any structure known to be contractile. The changes of calibre which occur in the vessels of the living web are in perfect harmony with this anatomical description; for while the arteries, even to their smallest branches, are sometimes constricted to absolute closure, and at other times widely dilated, the capillaries are never found to be entirely closed, nor to present any variations in diameter, which are not explicable by elasticity of their parietes.

The capillaries, though not contractile, are highly elastic, and by virtue of this property are capable of considerable variation in capacity, according to the distending force of the current of blood. Figs. 3 and 4 of Plate XLVII., traced with the cameya lucida, show, besides the pigment in two chromatophorous cells of the frog's foot, part of a capillary in nearly extreme conditions in point of calibre. In fig. 3 the vessel is about equal in diameter to the length of a red corpuscle, while in fig. 4 it is so narrow that the corpuscles in it are pinched transversely and elongated, When the capillaries are most distended, their parietes are much thinner than when shrunk to their smallest dimensions; an estimate may be formed of the difference by comparing the close proximity of the corpuscles to the outer bounding line of the vessel in fig. 3 with the considerable interval in fig. 4, that interval representing the apparent thickness of the wall of the vessel. It is to be observed that the frog had been killed in a manner involving considerable hemorrhage before fig. 4 was traced, so that the capillaries were then little, if at all, distended with blood. The thinness of the walls of the capillaries, as compared with the small arteries, is, doubtless, calculated to favour the mutual interchanges which must take place between the blood in them and the tissues in their vicinity. It is believed by some eminent authorities that mutual attractions and repulsions subsisting between the nutrient fluid and the tissues among which it flows, become a source of movement in the blood and assist its flow through the capillaries; while others regard the heart as the sole cause of the circulation: and the difference of opinion on this fundamental point in physiology involves discordance in pathological theory, for some who hold the former view consider the changes which occur in the circulation at the commencement of inflammation, to be principally owing to modifications of the 'vital' moving force. The view that such a cause of movement exists, has been supported partly by argument drawn from the phenomena of inflammation: but these, as we shall see, require a very different interpretation. It has also been based upon a supposed analogy between the circulation of the blood in the higher animals and certain movements observed to occur without any visible source of mechanical power in tubes and cells in the vegetable kingdom, and, as was thought, also in some of the lower forms of animal life: but though a resemblance may probably exist between some of these and the movements occurring in the processes of secretion and absorption and the circulation of nutrient fluid among the tissues of intercapillary spaces and non-vascular parts, the progress of modern discovery tends to show that the comparison is altogether inapplicable to the sanguiniferous system. It would, I think, be out of place to enter fully into this discussion on the present occasion, but my own experience with the frog leaves no doubt in my mind that in that animal contractions of the heart are the only cause of the circulation. I will content myself with mentioning two observations bearing upon this question. The first of these has reference to certain movements which occur for a considerable time after cessation of the heart's action, and which, though of trivial and uncertain character, have had much stress laid upon them in this discussion. I have ascertained by observations made in several different cases, that they are produced by occasional spontaneous contractions and relaxations of the arteries. These changes in the calibre of the vessels continue, even in an amputated limb, for days after severance from the body: I have repeatedly watched them taking place, and seen them give rise to the movement of the blood.

The other fact to which I will allude, appears to me to decide of itself the question at issue. Having occasion to examine, under chloroform, some very small frogs, measuring about an inch from the tip of the nose to the end of the coccyx, I found that the blood in the capillaries invariably flowed in a stream pulsating synchronously with the beats of the heart, which were visible through the parietes of the thorax; and however mildly the anesthetic was administered, the motion was commonly exceedingly slight between the pulses. Not unfrequently, although the arteries remained of full size, the blood moved in jerks, with considerable intervals of absolute stillness between the successive impulses which the contractions of the heart occasioned; yet no accumulation of corpuscles was produced in the capillaries, however long the animal was kept under observation. Had any other cause of motion than the action of the heart operated upon the blood, there must have been a continuous flow, however much accelerated at each pulse; for I must add, that there was nothing whatever of recoil after each onward movement, nor anything indicating obstruction to the progress of the blood.

Thus in these cases of intermitting capillary flow, it was matter of direct observation that the heart was the sole cause of the blood's motion; and as we know that in an animal under the influence of chloroform the changes of the blood from arterial to venous, and vice versa, continue to occur in the systemic and pulmonary capillaries, and as we have every reason to believe that the processes of nutrition in the different parts of the body go on then as usual, these cases appear to prove absolutely that the forces which are concerned in the mutual interchanges between the tissues and the nutrient fluid do not cause any movement whatever.

But even supposing that it were admitted, for the sake of argument, that the vital affinities do, under ordinary circumstances, cause some movement of the blood, but lose that power in an animal under chloroform, such an admission would hardly affect the discussion regarding the cause of stagnation in inflammation; for in a frog fully under the influence of the anesthetic, in which, as we have seen, the heart is the only cause of circulation, all the phenomena that result from irritation of the web take place precisely in the same manner as in one to which the narcotic has not been administered. The fact that the heart, even though much enfeebled by chloroform, is capable, unaided by any other force, of maintaining the circulation for an indefinite period without the occurrence of obstruction in the capillaries, or any undue accumulation of corpuscles in them, affords positive proof that any other cause of movement which may be conceived to exist when chloroform has not been given, must be altogether insignificant, and that the cessation of its operation does not give rise to stagnation of the blood.

The veins of the frog's web afford very little evidence of contractility; but a small amount of unstriped muscular tissue, transversely arranged, is distinctly to be seen in the larger venous branches; and on one occasion I observed a very considerable degree of local contraction, as measured from the outer borders of the external coat of a vein running through a small area which I had pinched forcibly with forceps. I have also seen one expand on sudden dilatation of the arteries of the web, so that its diameter increased from twelve to fourteen degrees of a micrometer; but this is perhaps explicable by elasticity?

It has been already mentioned that the arteries undergo spontaneous variations of' calibre. Such changes are constantly going on at varying intervals, there being nothing of a rhythmical character about them. A struggle on the part of the animal is generally accompanied by a very considerable constriction of the arteries, and sometimes by absolute closure of them. The contraction usually begins a very short time before the motions of the body, so that the struggle can commonly be predicted by the appearance of the vessels; and dilatation occurs when the creature becomes quiet. Hence the changes of calibre are evidently under the control of the nerves. An account of an inquiry into the parts of the nervous system by which this control is exercised, will be found at p. 607 of this volume; and from the experiments there recorded, it will be seen that either extreme constriction or full dilatation of the arteries of the web may be induced at pleasure, by operating upon the spinal cord. A very good opportunity is thus afforded for studying the effects produced upon the capillary circulation by changes of calibre in the arteries, without employing any means acting directly upon the foot. This is a matter of very great importance, for applications made to the web for the purpose of inducing alterations in the dimensions of the vessels, give rise at the same time to other consequences of irritation, which complicate such experiments in a most deceptive manner, so as to have misled, as I believe, some of the best observers who have devoted attention to this subject.

The following account embodies the results of numerous observations in which this source of fallacy was carefully avoided, the variations in the calibre of the vessels being generally either induced by operations on the cord, or else such as occurred spontaneously.

In a perfectly healthy state of the web with the heart beating powerfully, when the arteries are of about medium width, the current of blood in them is so rapid that the individual corpuscles cannot be discerned; but in the capillaries, whose aggregate calibre is very much greater than that of the arterial trunk which feeds them, the flow is so much slower that they can be pretty clearly distinguished. When the arteries are fully dilated, if the heart continues to act with the same energy, the blood appears to move as rapidly in them as before, though of course In much larger quantity; while in the capillaries the flow is extremely accelerated, so that it becomes as impossible to see the blood-corpuscles in them as in the arteries. On the other hand, when the arteries are considerably constricted, the blood moves more slowly through the capillaries than when the tubes of supply are of medium size, and at the same time the narrowed arteries appear to filter the blood more or less of corpuscles, which are found in smaller numbers in proportion to the liquor sanguinis in the capillaries: and if the constriction of the arteries is sufficiently great, the web is rendered quite pale in consequence of the small number of corpuscles in it, which nevertheless continue to move among the tortuous capillaries, producing in the field of the microscope an appearance something like that of a few flies playing about in a room. Finally, if the arteries are completely constricted, all appearance of flow in the capillaries vanishes, and the web has a wholly exsanguine aspect. Under these circumstances, even the veins, though still of large calibre, may contain little besides colourless liquor sanguinis, which has continued to ooze through the contracted arteries when the corpuscles have been completely arrested; and so inconspicuous do the veins become in consequence of this change in the quality of their contents, that it may be extremely difficult to distinguish them from other tissues; the appearance of the web on superficial observation being as if it possessed no blood-vessels at all. This remarkable condition, which, so far as I know, has not been before described, may last for several minutes in consequence of irritation of the cord, and in one case I observed it occur spontaneously, and continue for five minutes together. It appears to be comparable to the dead whiteness of the human fingers when benumbed with cold, or the perfect pallor of the cheek in faintness; while blushing is no doubt caused by full dilatation of the arteries.

Such, according to my experience, are the effects produced upon the circulation by changes of calibre in the vessels of a perfectly healthy web. The arteries regulate by their contractility the amount of blood transmitted in a given time through the capillaries, but neither full dilatation, extreme constriction, nor any intermediate state of the former is capable *per se* of producing accumulation of corpuscles in the latter.

SECTION III: *On the Effects of Irritants upon the Circulation.*

It is well known that the application of an irritant substance to the web of the frog's foot is followed by changes of calibre in the blood-vessels, and also by an abnormal accumulation within them of the corpuscular elements of the blood. The first experiments which I performed upon the frog were directed to the solution of the much-debated question, whether or no the latter were a mere consequence of the former; and although it has, I think, been sufficiently shown at the conclusion of the last section that such cannot be the case, yet it will be well to allude shortly to these experiments on account of their further bearing upon the subject of this inquiry.

It occurred to me, that if, instead of the powerful irritants commonly used in these investigations, some exceedingly mild stimulant were employed, the changes in the calibre of the vessels might perhaps be produced without concomitant alterations of the blood. The material which appeared most suitable for this purpose was warm water, which is known to cause, in the human subject, increased redness without inflammation of the part to which it is applied.

Accordingly, in September 1855 I endeavoured to ascertain its effects upon the frog. In most of the experiments, the foot of the animal being stretched under the microscope upon a glass plate somewhat inclined, so that any fluid upon it might run off quickly, an assistant threw a stream of water of known temperature upon it by means of a syringe, the eye of the observer being kept over the microscope, which was provided with a micrometer in its eyepiece. In this way the effects produced by the water could be seen almost immediately after it had ceased to play upon the web, and the changes of calibre in any artery selected for observation were noted with precision. It was found that the result of the warm application was constriction of the arteries to absolute closure, generally lasting for several seconds, and then giving place to dilatation beyond their original dimensions, to which they afterwards gradually returned. The dilatation differed in different instances, being generally more decided and more permanent when the water was hotter and longer applied In one case, water at 100' thrown upon the web for a brief period caused constriction for a few seconds in the artery under observation, followed by dilatation. While the vessels were still above their usual calibre, more water of the same temperature was applied as before, and again induced contraction followed by abnormal dilatation, which was again made to give place to constriction by a third similar application: the experiments were repeated within a few seconds of each other.

When water not higher in temperature than from 110" to 140' was thrown for not longer than a second or two upon a perfectly healthy web, the changes above described in the diameter of the arteries produced effects upon the flow of blood through the capillaries, precisely similar to those mentioned at the conclusion of the last section. Thus in one such case the constriction of an artery lasted for several seconds, and was in the first instance so tight as to prevent any flow in the field of capillaries supplied by it; then relaxing slightly, it allowed single corpuscles to pass along it with great difficulty, so that the blood became almost entirely filtered of its particles, and at the same time the force of the heart being to a great extent taken off from the elastic capillaries, liquor sanguinis almost destitute of corpuscles flowed in slow pulsating streams along the veins: finally, the dilatation becoming complete, blood of ordinary appearance rushed through with great rapidity.

If, however, such experiments had been several times repeated upon the same foot, and more especially if the warm water had acted for longer periods, another class of symptoms began to show themselves; the corpuscles passing on less freely than the liquor sanguinis through the capillaries, and lagging behind so as to accumulate in abnormal proportion to the plasma, and stagnating completely when the force of the heart was partially taken off through contraction of the arteries, though passing on again when the vessels dilated Thus in one case an artery under observation measuring 2" (degrees of the micrometer), the blood was flowing in all the capillaries supplied by it, though containings very abnormal amount of corpuscles. After a few minutes, the vessel contracted spontaneously to 1 r, and though this was only about a medium width, the flow of the blood became much retarded in the capillaries, and in one of them ceased almost entirely. Water of 115 degrees Fahrenheit was thrown upon the web, the calibre of the artery was raised to above 2 degrees, and the flow was resumed in all the capillaries. A few minutes later the vessel again contracted spontaneously to 1½ degrees when stagnation of the blood became nearly complete in a few of the capillaries. Water at 120' was then applied and caused constriction to a further degree, followed by dilatation to above 2': during the constriction, the blood scarcely moved at all in the capillaries, but on the occurrence of the dilatation it again flowed in all of them.

If the applications were still further continued, the red discs became more and more closely packed, till at last they were crammed together so as to produce a uniform crimson mass, unaffected by the heart even in the widest state of the arteries.

It was perfectly clear that in these experiments the stagnation of the blood depended on something more than mere contraction of the arteries; and it also appeared impossible to account for it satisfactorily as a result of their dilatation. That inflammatory stasis might occur independently of alteration in the calibre of the vessels, was also shown by an experiment with capsicum made at this period. A morsel of this substance having been placed upon the middle of a web in which the circulation was going on in perfect health and with unusual rapidity, the effect was great accumulation of corpuscles in two or three capillaries for a very short distance round the spot where the capsicum lay, unaccompanied by any change in the vascular dimensions.

Chloroform proved to be an agent which very readily induced stagnation when locally applied; and when it was administered in the usual way by inhalation for the purpose of performing experiments with warm water, it was found necessary to protect the webs carefully from its vapour, which otherwise produced the same appearances of congestion as the hot application. In one instance in which a small quantity of the liquid had been applied to the web, I saw the red corpuscles adhering to one another by their flat surfaces, in a manner not seen in the healthy condition, and exactly as described by Mr. WHARTON JONES to take place after the application of a strong solution of salt; but from the very slight tendency of chloroform to mix with water, it was impossible to believe that it had operated by way of exosmose, as was supposed by the authority just named to be the case with the saline solution.

From the facts above mentioned, I became convinced that no satisfactory explanation had as yet been given of the obstruction experienced by the blood-corpuscles in the vessels of an inflamed part, and in September 1856 I again continued the investigation. Mustard being admitted to produce inflammation in any part of the human body to which it is applied, and also not appearing likely to act by way of exosmose, I selected it as a suitable irritant, and in order to study its effects accurately, placed a small portion of its moistened flour, about a line in diameter, upon the middle of the web of a large frog under chloroform. After a while, thinking that I saw stagnation in a capillary just at the margin of the mustard, I removed the latter with a camel's-hair brush, and was surprised to find that throughout the whole area on which it had lain, the capillaries were crammed with either stagnant or very slowly moving red corpuscles. The limits of the part so affected corresponded exactly with the extent of the application of the mustard, although the capillaries of adjoining parts were fed and drained by the same arteries and veins.

On the 3rd of October I made another similar experiment, selecting a part of the web where a considerable artery divided into small branches. Before applying the irritant, I had ascertained that the artery running through the area measured 6g of an eyepiece micrometer, while a large vein near it had a diameter of 12". About half a minute after the application of the mustard, when I first looked through the microscope, the arteries of the web generally were much dilated, and the flow, which had before been somewhat languid, was rapid in all its capillaries. The opacity of the mustard prevented the vessels beneath it from being observed, but at a short distance from its edge the artery measured 10" and the vein 14". In a few minutes the capillaries seen beneath the extreme margin of the mustard, which was slightly transparent, were observed to be of crimson colour, in consequence of their containing closely-crammed corpuscles, some of which were still moving, while others were motionless. On the application of a higher power, the continuations of these capillaries immediately exterior to the mustard showed, many of them, red corpuscles sticking to their walls, and more or less obstructing the progress of the blood through them.

In the accompanying sketch of the vessels at one part, together with those corpuscles which, were motionless in them, M represents the edge of the mustard, *a* a capillary partly overlaid by the mustard and crammed with stagnant corpuscles, 6 a capillary with red discs adhering to its internal surface, but still transmitting blood, while further from the mustard all the corpuscles were in motion, and consequently none appear in the drawing; *c* was a rouleau of red corpuscles projecting from a stagnant mass into the vein V, through which the blood was flowing rapidly; yet the rouleau, though its free end was moved to and fro by the current, was prevented by the mutual adhesiveness of its corpuscles from being broken up or detached. Thus it was evident that in the capillaries of the space covered by the mustard, the red corpuscles had an abnormal tendency to adhere both to the walls of the vessels and to one another, and were on this account accumulating and sticking within them, while almost immediately outside the mustard, the blood in the capillaries presented the same appearance as in other parts of the web. This effect was independent of changes in the calibre of the vessels, for any results of alteration in the size of the artery under the mustard must have been shared by the surrounding capillaries, which also derived their blood chiefly from it; and that the vessel was dilated to the same degree there as elsewhere, was shown by the fact, that its branches continued throughout the experiment to transmit full streams of blood after emerging from beneath the opaque mass. I also measured some capillaries by micrometer before the application of the mustard, and again after it had caused stagnation in them, and found that their dimensions remained the same.

The precise limitation of the effect produced upon the blood in these two experiments to the area covered by the mustard, showed that it was the result of a direct action of the irritant either upon the blood that flowed beneath it, or upon the tissues of the part of the web on which it lay, the blood being in the latter case affected secondarily. I made several experiments to determine whether the adhesiveness of the corpuscles in blood out of the body was increased by contact with, or vicinity to mustard, placing minute portions of it between plates of glass, and shedding a drop of blood from a frog, so that it might run in between the plates, and watching the result. I could, however, detect no evidence of such change in the corpuscles as I was seeking; whence I inferred that the blood had been only affected secondarily to the tissues in the two mustard experiments.

A careful study of the effects produced by the local application of chloroform to the web, confirmed in every respect the conclusions previously arrived at. If, while the eye of the observer is over the microscope, a minute drop of this liquid is placed with a camel's-hair brush upon the part in the field of view, it evaporates in perhaps two or three seconds; and if the web be dry, the time of its disappearance can be distinctly seen. Yet though it has so short a time to act, it produces so powerful an effect upon the part, that the red corpuscles immediately experience obstruction to their progress, and move too slowly in abnormal numbers through the capillaries, which perhaps become entirely clogged with them; the arteries meanwhile being in the state best adapted for easy transmission of the blood, i.e. full dilatation. In one such experiment I saw a few corpuscles sticking together in a capillary and moving with difficulty, from evident tendency to adhere to its parietes, their number gradually becoming augmented by the adhesion of others that followed, till the mass grew so large as to fill the vessel for some distance, when it finally stopped. In another case, the circulation being perfectly natural in the web, and the corpuscles moving on at slight intervals with no tendency to adhere, on a drop of chloroform being applied, I saw the very same corpuscles instantly become checked in their progress by sticking to each other and to the capillary walls, and move on slowly in masses with considerable intervals. Thus the nature of the effect produced upon the red corpuscles of the blood when chloroform is applied to the web is the same as that caused by mustard, viz. an abnormal degree of adhesiveness; whereas the earliest evidence of the direct action of chloroform on blood out of the body is the loss of the adhesive property of the red discs, as has been mentioned in Section I. That the effect on the blood within the vessels of a part inflamed by chloroform is secondary to a change in the tissues is further proved by the circumstance, that abnormal accumulation of slowly moving corpuscles may last for hours together without stagnation, as a consequence of the application of this irritant for an extremely brief period. Long after all the blood which could possibly have been directly acted on by the chloroform has left the vessels, successive fresh portions continue to experience precisely similar changes in passing through the irritated area.

Heat produces similar effects. If the foot of a frog which is under the influence of chloroform be covered entirely with wet lint, except a small area of one of the webs, and a red-hot cautery iron be held for a few seconds about half an inch above the exposed part, inflammation will be excited in the area in proportion to the time of the action of the dry heat upon it; but on removal of the lint, the circulation will be found perfectly healthy in the surrounding parts. In the severer cases stagnation is universal in the exposed area, and the epidermis becomes eventually raised by the exudation of serum beneath it; but in milder instances nothing more than accumulation of slowly-moving corpuscles is produced, and I have observed this state of the part to continue for hours after the heat was applied. Here again the effect on the blood was obviously not due to the direct action of the heat upon it, but to some changes which it had effected in the tissues of the part on which it had acted. Evidence of the same kind, but still more conclusive, is derived from the effects of mechanical irritation, where the agency is free from all objection of possible chemical action on the blood. The method adopted was that of compressing a small part of the middle of the web between little pads of soft material attached to the ends of the blades of a pair of surgical dressing forceps, by which the degree of pressure could be regulated at will. The results of this treatment were identical with those of heat, as just described. If the pressure was not made too severe, no mechanical obstruction was produced in the vessels, which nevertheless became loaded with slowly-moving or stagnant corpuscles; and on one occasion I observed the capillaries of an area which had been pinched, still transmitting languid streams of blood containing great excess of corpuscles several days after the injury had been inflicted, while in the surrounding parts the circulation continued perfectly healthy. Mechanical violence, like heat, chloroform and mustard, had effected an alteration in the tissues on which it operated, in consequence of which the blood in their vicinity assumed abnormal characters; and many other facts of similar nature might be added, if necessary, to show that this is the course always followed when accumulation of corpuscles in the vessels is induced by the action of irritants.

In discussions regarding the causes of the phenomena of inflammation seen in the frog's web, the great difficulty has hitherto been to account for the puzzling fact, that while the arteries still retain that state of enlarged calibre which is best adapted for easy transmission of the blood, its accelerated movement comes to give place to unnatural retardation and ultimate stagnation. Accordingly, various theories, mechanical, chemical and vital, have been proposed to explain the transition from "determination of blood," as the condition of dilatation of the arteries with increased flow through the capillaries has been termed, to inflammatory congestion, as the accumulation of corpuscles in the vessels may perhaps be most fitly designated. But the second simple experiment with mustard, to which I would again direct the attention of the reader, proves in a very beautiful manner that these two results of irritation are totally distinct in nature and independent in cause. The dilatation of the arteries, it will be remembered, affected not only the part on which the mustard lay, but also all the rest of the web, showing that it was developed indirectly through the medium of the nervous system; whereas the accumulation of the blood-corpuscles in the vessels below the mustard was, as we have seen, the result of the direct action of the irritant upon the tissues. The arterial dilatation in the web generally led to no changes in the quality of the blood, which, though the experiment was continued for some hours, retained to the last its natural characters, just as would have been the case had the enlargement of the vessels depended on an operation performed upon the spinal cord. The accumulation of corpuscles, on the other hand, implied an alteration in the properties of the blood, viz. an abnormal adhesiveness in the red discs. Determination of blood is thus a purely functional phenomenon, and, like a blush upon the cheek, becomes obliterated after death by the post-mortem contractions of the vessels: inflammatory congestion, on the contrary, is the first evidence of organic lesion, and declares itself as distinctly in the dead as in the living, being the most important if not the only sign of the early stages of inflammation discoverable on dissection., as for instance in the case of incipient meningitis mentioned in the Introduction to this paper.

Although determination of blood, as met with in the frog, is thus entirely independent of inflammatory congestion, yet it is of great interest with reference to human inflammation. Dilatation of the arteries is now generally admitted to be the result of the relaxation of their muscular fibres; and that it is a purely passive phenomenon, seems to be absolutely demonstrated by the fact which I have pointed out elsewhere, that after the vessels have been liberated from the control of the nervous system by removal of the spinal cord, they dilate fully if the heart continues to act sufficiently powerfully to distend them with blood, but not otherwise. Recent physiological discovery has shown that the arteries are not singular in being thrown into a state of muscular relaxation through irritation of the parts of the nervous system connected with them, the same being the case with the heart, the intestines, and apparently also with other hollow viscera. In a preliminary account of an inquiry into the functions of the visceral nerves, published in the 'Proceedings' of this Society, I have given some notice of experiments which seem to show that in the case of the viscera alluded to, the state of relaxation under such circumstances is the result of the more energetic operation of nerves, which, when working more mildly, increase the muscular action of the same organs; the functions of the ganglia specially concerned in regulating the movements of the viscera being exalted by gentle stimulation on the part of the afferent nerves connected with them, but depressed by stronger excitation. In that paper the opinion was expressed, that the same explanation probably applies to the relaxation of the arteries, in consequence of nervous irritation; the general impression conveyed by the experiments with warm water above related being that arterial contraction was most apt to show itself when the degree of irritation was least, while dilatation was most marked when the stimulus was strongest. I have lately seen a striking illustration of this principle in a very simple experiment, which I was induced to make in consequence of reading a paper recently published by a French author, M. J. MAREY. If a bluntpointed instrument, such as the end of a pair of dissecting forceps, is drawn with gentle pressure along the back of the hand while it is in a state of moderate redness, the blood being driven out of the vessels, a pale streak results, which immediately disappears, in consequence of the return of the blood into the part. In a few seconds, however, a pale stripe, towards a quarter of an inch in breadth, becomes developed at each side of the line along which the instrument passed, that line having now assumed a red colour, if the pressure employed was at all forcible. This is M. MARE's experiment; and there can be no doubt that his interpretation of the secondary paleness is correct, viz. that it depends on reflex arterial contraction. The red line, when it occurs, is evidently due to the direct action of the pressure upon the tissues, being, as M. MAREY correctly states, exactly of the same breadth as the instrument used. But I find that if the pressure be made with considerably greater force, so as to be positively painful, while the first white streak appears as before in consequence of the blood being dispelled from the vessels, the secondary paleness does not occur, but, on the contrary, a patch of the adjacent skin, extending for perhaps half an inch on each side, assumes abnormal redness, which lasts for a longer time than the paleness to which the other experiment gives rise. Here, the irritation being severe, the blood vessels are thrown through the medium of the nervous system into a state of muscular relaxation, instead of the contraction which is induced by a more gentle application of the same stimulus.

To return to the consideration of inflammatory congestion. Further light was thrown upon the condition of the blood in the vessels of an irritated part by a series of observations made when the circulation had been arrested by amputation of the limb, or by a ligature round the thigh. This field of inquiry was unexpectedly opened during the course of an experiment made with a view to ascertaining the effects produced by an irritant upon the pigmentary system independently of the circulation, as will be described in the next section. On the 13th of October 1856, a frog having been killed by destruction of the brain, the soft parts of one of the thighs were divided to the bone, and a small piece of mustard was placed on one of the webs of that foot. An hour afterwards, on removing the mustard, I saw to my great surprise that the small area on which it had lain was red to the naked eye, and that its capillaries, examined microscopically, contained abundance of closely-packed corpuscles, while in surrounding parts the blood was in the same condition as before the experiment, via. of pretty healthy aspect. In other words, well-marked inflammatory congestion had been produced by the mustard, and I afterwards found that the same thing occurred in a limb completely severed from the body.

This fact of course completely eliminated variations in the calibre of the vessels and consequent changes in the circulation from among the causes of congestion, and demonstrated conclusively its independence of the central organs of the nervous system. Further, it presented a very good opportunity for studying the state of the blood in healthy and inflamed parts, unaccompanied by the effects of rapid movement. In subsequent similar experiments, it was found that the corpuscles were not brought to the irritated area by anything that indicated a mutual attraction between the former and. the latter, but were simply carried along by slight accidental movements of the blood, such as are caused by post-mortem contractions of the arteries, and instead of moving with facility, as in other parts, stuck when they arrived in the vessels of the area, in consequence of undue adhesiveness. The accumulation of the corpuscles was never to such an extent as in cases in which the heart was driving the blood through the part, but it affected the arterial and venous branches as well as the capillaries. Thus, if a large vein happened to run through the spot upon which the mustard mas placed, it became in time choked with a crimson mass of corpuscles in that part of its extent which lay beneath the mustard; but immediately beyond, in both directions, the blood in it contained no more than the usual proportion of corpuscles, or sometimes considerably less; and these moved freely to and fro when the web was touched, whereas those within the area remained fixed. This proved that the cause of the accumulation of the corpuscles did not reside specially in the capillaries, and also showed distinctly that it could not be explained by mere abnormal adhesiveness of the vascular parietes, which was, I understand, the view entertained by the late Dr. MARSHALL HALL; for supposing the walls of the vessels to experience such a change, which seems by no means improbable, this could only lead to encrusting of the lining membrane of such a vein with adhering corpuscles, and not to the occupation of its whole calibre by them, as took place in these cases, unless the corpuscles were themselves also abnormally adhesive.

Another important fact which was brought out by this class of experiments is, that mere quiescence of the blood in the vessels of a healthy part fails to induce aggregation of the red corpuscles, such as occurs in blood outside the body. In the parts which had not been subjected to irritation, the corpuscles exhibited no trace of adhesiveness; and though completely at rest, they were nowhere to be seen grouped together, surface to surface, although in the larger vessels there was abundant space for the occurrence of this phenomenon, which invariably presents itself in freshly drawn frog's blood examined between plates of glass in a sufficiently thick film. On one occasion, when examining the tissues of the web of a frog under chloroform, the limb being kept steady by a string tied tightly round the thigh, so as completely to arrest the circulation, I was particularly struck with the total absence of adhesiveness in the red corpuscles; so much so, that, as the foot had been kept moist without circulation for about three hours, I suspected that it must have imbibed water, which, when mixed with blood outside the body, destroys altogether the adhesiveness of the red corpuscles. This, however, proved to be a mistake; for, having occasion to administer more chloroform, 1 applied it on a piece of lint of considerable size without taking the usual precaution of protecting the foot from the vapour, and left it so for about a quarter of an hour. On re-examination of the web, the red corpuscles were found to possess much mutual adhesiveness, and in the larger vessels were grouped together into masses, with considerable spaces of clear liquor sanguinis, just as in the best-marked forms of aggregation in frog's blood outside the body. One of these masses was drawn by camera lucida, and is represented in the sketch at page 648, along with the outline of the vessel in which it lay. I afterwards purposely induced a similar change in the blood within the vessels of an amputated limb by means of mustard. Having ascertained that the red corpuscles, though they had been long at rest, were perfectly free from the slightest tendency to aggregation, I suspended, at a little distance from the web, a piece of lint smeared with freshly prepared mustard, so that the pungent vapour of the volatile oil might play upon it; and left it so for about a quarter of an hour, when I found the red discs aggregated, as usually seen in frog's blood outside the body. I then shed some blood from the other leg between two plates of glass, and on carefully sketching and comparing the groups of corpuscles in this specimen and those within the vessels of the irritated webs, found that their characters were precisely similar". These are examples of what very numerous observations have tended to establish, namely, that on the one hand the red corpuscles in the vessels of a perfectly healthy part are free from adhesiveness; and on the other hand, the adhesiveness which they acquire in inflammatory congestion, though varying in proportion to the degree of irritation, is never greater than occurs in the blood of a healthy part when withdrawn from the body.

These conclusions, if correct, represent cardinal truths, both in physiology and pathology, implying relations of the tissues to the blood both in health and in disease, such as have never before been demonstrated, or, I believe, even suspected. I was therefore anxious to submit them to further test, particularly as it is by no means easy to estimate the precise degree of adhesiveness possessed by the red corpuscles within the vessels; and it occurred to me that one means of' doing this would be to compare specimens of blood shed from inflamed and healthy parts of the same individual; for if my deductions were sound, the adhesiveness of the red corpuscles ought to be neither more nor less in the one case than in the other.

With this view I made the following experiments. Having carefully examined the blood of a large frog, drawn from a subcutaneous vein of the abdomen, so as to become quite familiar with the appearance of its corpuscles, I applied mustard to the whole surface of one foot till inflammatory congestion had been fully developed in it, and then, amputating both feet at the ankle-joint, squeezed out blood from each upon a glass plate, and carefully examined both specimens, without being able to detect the slightest difference between them. The other experiments with this object were performed on the human subject. In one of these I applied a portion of moistened mustard to the dorsal aspect of the last phalanx of one of my fingers, and retained it there for five hours, with the exception of occasional removal for the purpose of drawing blood for examination. By the conclusion of the time mentioned, the skin on which the mustard had been placed was in a very decided state of inflammation, being red, swollen and painful, and the redness at one spot disappearing imperfectly on pressure, and returning languidly after its removal. A very minute drop of blood drawn with a fine needle from the surface of the most inflamed part was then compared with a drop of similar size from another finger, but no difference could be detected between them, nor had any been observed in previous similar comparisons. On another occasion, a friend of mine suffering from intense inflammation of the back of the hand, in consequence of the irritation of offensive pus, permitted me to take blood with a needle from the most severely affected part, and also from one of the fingers, which was healthy. I compared drops from the two sources several times very carefully with each other by means of the microscope, but could discover no difference between them in the adhesiveness of their corpuscles; as indicated by the time of formation of the rouleaux, their mode of grouping, and the tenacity with which the discs composing them adhered when they were stretched. The results of these experiments appear decidedly confirmatory of the conclusion with reference to which they were instituted.

No mention has been hitherto made of the appearance presented by the colourless corpuscles in an irritated part. It is well known that their numbers, in proportion to the red ones, vary very much in different frogs, and it so happened that in the two on which the first mustard experiments were performed they showed themselves but little; nor are they at all conspicuous when the circulation has been arrested by ligature; but in most cases in which irritation is applied to the web while the blood is circulating through it, one of the earliest abnormal appearances is that of white corpuscles adhering in large numbers to the walls of arteries, capillaries and veins, as first described and accurately figured by Dr. WILLIAMS. This remarkable phenomenon, though of itself clear proof of an alteration in the properties of the blood in an irritated part, has, strangely enough, attracted little attention from other observers. It is evidently analogous to the change which the red discs experience under similar circumstances. I find that the account commonly given of the white corpuscles in circulation in the vessels of the frog's web, viz. that they may be seen rolling slowly along the walls of the arteries and veins, and sometimes sticking to them, though intended to apply to the state of health?, really describes a condition of a slight amount of irritation, such as is exceedingly apt to be induced by a variety of causes. In perfect health the colourless corpuscles are as free from adhesiveness within the vessels as the red discs, but like them assume that property in a degree proportionate to the amount of irritation to which the part has been subjected. When the irritation has been very slight, the white corpuscles, which are susceptible of much greater adhesiveness than the red (as we learn from examining blood outside the body), acquire some tendency to stick to the vascular parietes, while the red discs still move on in a manner generally regarded as consistent with health, though really lagging slightly behind the liquor sanguinis, and consequently presenting themselves in somewhat abnormal proportion. I have often observed the complete absence of adhesiveness of the white corpuscles within the vessels in health, and have also watched them gradually assume a tendency to adhere, in consequence of repeated mild applications of chloroform to a web in which they previously exhibited no such disposition whatever. As the irritation increases, the vessels become crusted with them often to a remarkable degree, and occasionally large, colourless, agglomerated masses of them, just such as are seen in blood drawn from the body, may be observed to roll along the large veins among the slowly lnoving and very numerous red discs. I once watched the formation of one of these masses as a delta-like accumulation at the place where a considerable venous branch opened into a main trunk, the calibre of which was nearly entirely occupied by it before it was swept away by the current. As a general rule, the white corpuscles when adhering do not arrest the progress of the red ones, which are often seen to pass through very small intervals among the colourless masses; not unfrequently, however, red corpuscles are stopped in their course and adhere among the white ones, and sometimes, especially in young frogs, capillaries become obstructed throughout their entire length by white corpuscles alone, and when this is the case, they are apt to escape notice from the inconspicuous character of their contents.

The adhesiveness of the white corpuscles, as of the red ones, is limited to the part irritated. A very good example of this presented itself on one occasion when a minute drop of chloroform was applied to a small part of a healthy web so as to induce full dilatation of the arteries and great excess of corpuscles, but without absolute stagnation. It happened that the part affected was supplied with blood by the branches coming from one side of a principal artery; the main trunk being seated just about the limit between the irritated area and the healthy region, the adjacent part of which received supply from the branches of the vessel on the other side. The latter showed no appearance of adhering white corpuscles, nor did the capillaries which were fed by them; but those of the irritated part, though springing from the same trunk, mere remarkably encrusted. with them from their origin to their minutest ramifications within the area, while the capillaries and veins in the same part were similarly affected. This striking appearance continued for hours after the chloroform had been applied, successive fully formed white corpuscles adhering as they flowed in from the trunk, being evidently affected secondarily to the change induced by the chloroform in the tissues of the web.

Thus the affection of the white corpuscles of the blood in an irritated part is in all respects strictly parallel to that of the red discs, while the greater adhesiveness of which the former are capable, renders the facts regarding them more obvious and unmistakable.

Being desirous to verify the results derived from the frog by observations upon mammalia, in which the aggregation of the red corpuscles assumes a much more striking appearance, I examined the wings of two small bats. In the first specimen, the corpuscles, both red and white, exhibited decided adhesiveness within the vessels, the web being apparently in a state of irritation from injuries which the animal had sustained. In the other there was also some adhesiveness in the part that first met my eye, the red discs tending to aggregate into rouleaux, and giving a lumpy aspect to the somewhat dark streams in the larger vessels: but turning to another place, I found the blood there of pale tint and perfectly homogeneous aspect; nor could I detect by a careful search any evidence of a tendency on the part of the white corpuscles to stick to the vascular parietes. It happened that there was complete absence of flow in one artery and concomitant vein of considerable size, yet not a rouleau was to be seen either in them or in any of their branches. On the contraly, the red discs lay at about equal distances from each other, uniformly distributed throughout the calibre of the vessels; and this state of things remained unchanged during about a quarter of an hour, in which I continued to observe thein in their perfectly quiescent condition. On examination of some blood from the heart of this bat shortly after, the red corpuscles exhibited a very remarkable degree of adhesiveness, such as I had never seen in human bloodYkp, resenting a glaring contrast with their state within the vesselsf.

Thus we may, I think, regard it as fully established, that, in mammalia as well as in amphibia, both the red discs and the colourless globules of the blood are completely free from adhesiveness within the vesscls of a perfectly healthy part, but that when the tissues have suffered from irritation, both kinds of corpuscles assume, in proportion to the severity of the affection, a degree of that tendency to stick to one another and to neighbouring objects which they possess when withdrawn from the body, and consequently experience obstruction to their progress through the minute vessels.

And here I cannot avoid remarking, that this principle explains, if it does not altogether reconcile, the discordant opinions of physiologists rcgarding the causes of the circulation.

It shows that while there is, as we have before seen, strong ground for agreeing with those who hold that the flow of the blood is due simply to the contractions of the heart, aided, in animals with valved veins, by the actions of the muscles, the respiratory movements, and, in the case of the bat's wing, by rhythmical venous contractions; yet there is also much truth in the view of those who maintain that the tissues of a part, independently of any change of calibre in the vessels, exercise a great influence upon the progress of the blood through the capillaries. For though the tissues do not, as has been hitherto supposed by the latter class of authorities, actively promote the circulation, yet their healthy condition is none the less necessary to it, being essential to the fitness of the blood for transmission by the heart through the minute vessels.

It is an interesting question, whether the freedom of the corpuscles from adhesiveness in health is due to some active operation of the tissues upon the vital fluid, or whether their adhesiveness in an inflamed part or outside the body is the result of a prejudicial influence exerted upon the blood by the irritated tissues, or by the objects of the external world with which it comes in contact when shed. The fact that the nonadhesiveness of the corpuscles within the vessels continues in an amputated limb, shows that it is independent of the central organs of the nervous system, and probably too of any nutritive actions going on in the tissues. Also, if the latter were concerned in its production, we should expect to find the corpuscles adhesive in the large arteries and veins of the webs, since it is doubtless chiefly in the capillaries that the mutual interchanges take place between the blood and the solid elements of the body. It may be difficult to obtain further evidence upon this point, but some light may be thrown upon it by the consideration of the causes of the coagulation of the blood, which seems to be a closely allied subject.

I have shown elsewhere, that in mamrnalia, as well as in amphibia, the blood remains fluid for days in the veins of an amputated healthy limb, though retaining its property of coagulating when shed Its fluidity within the vessels is unaffected by free admixture of the atmosphere with it. For example, seven hours after injecting air into the veins of an amputated sheep's foot, I found the frothy mixture contained in the vessels still quite fluid; and the blood which formed the bubbles, coagulated when shed. Again, a human leg having been amputated above the knee, I pressed out the blood from about an inch of the open mouth of the popliteal vein, and covered the raw surface lightly with a damp cloth, so as to guard against drying of the blood, or of the walls of the vessel in contact with it, After the lapse of twenty-four hours, the vessel was still patulous; but the blood, though it had been so long freely exposed to the influence of the air, continued perfectly fluid. Further, if a vein in an amputated sheep's foot is simply wounded, no clot forms except at the seat of wound. If, however, a portion of any ordinary solid matter, such as a fragment of glass, a bit of clean wax, a hair, a needle, or a piece of fine silver wire, be introduced into such a vein, a deposit of fibrine takes place after some minutes upon the foreign body, followed by coagulation of the blood in that particular part of the vessel; the coagulum, however, never adhering to the vein, except at the lips of the wound. This shows that an ordinary solid possesses an attraction for the particles of the fibrine, such as is not exercised by the walls of the vessels; or, in other words, that the vascular parietes differ from all ordinary solid substances in being destitute of attraction for that element of the liquor sanguinis.

The blood-vessels are not the only constituents of the animal body which have these remarkable relations to the blood. If the integument of a sheep's foot be partially reflected, and one of the subcutaneous veins immediately wounded, so as to let sorrle blood run into the angle between the skill and the rest of the limb, before any drying of the tissues has occurred, care being taken that no hairs or other solid matters have been introduced, this blood will remain in whole or in part fluid for half an hour or more; whereas, if blood from the same vessel be placed in contact with any ordinary solid, whether on the foot or elsewhere, it will coagulate in perhaps five minutes. This is sufficient proof that the subcutaneous cellular tissue resembles the lining membrane of the vessels in its conduct towards the blood. The long time during which blood has been observed to remain fluid but coagulable in the tunica vaginalis, seems to show that serous membranes are similarly circumstanced; and it appears probable that the same may be the case with other tissues.

But though some of the facts above mentioned furnish clear evidence that ordinary solid matter induces coagulation by an attractive agency, it by no means follows that the tissues are necessarily merely neutral in their conduct towards the blood in this matter. It is quite possible that they may exert an active influence upon it, in consequence of which the particles of fibrine may experience a mutual repulsion, in the same way as would seem to be the case with the pigment-granules of the chromatophorous cells of the frog during the process of diffusion. Indeed some such hypothesis seems almost necessary in order to explain the remarkable fact, that the blood coagulates within a few hours of death in the cavities of the heart and great venous trunks, though it retains its fluidity for days in the smaller vessels. Thus in the human subject twenty-four hours after death 7 have found clots in the heart and larger veins, including the upper parts of the axillary and femoral trunks, but fluid blood in the lower parts of those vessels and all their branches in the limbs. It seemed possible at first that this difference might depend on the position of the great vessels in the thorax and abdomen, where decomposition begins earlier than in the limbs. But this proved not to be the case; for in a horse twelve hours after it had been killed, I found the blood fluid in the intercostal and small cardiac veins, though coagulated in the vena cava and the coronary vein of the heart, which is in that animal of very large size. There being no reason to suppose the walls of the larger vessels differently constituted from those of the smaller ones, or more liable to undergo post mortem changes, the natural interpretation of these facts seems to be that the blood has, even within the body, a certain tendency to coagulation, counteracted by an influence exerted upon it by the containing tissues, which, operating to less advantage the larger the mass of the fluid acted on, fail, at least after death, to prevent it from following its natural course in vessels of a certain magnitude. Again, if we suppose that the tissues are merely passive with regard to the blood, it seems difficult to understand the rapid solidification of a large quantity shed into a cup. For we have seen that mere exposure to the atmosphere will not account for the fact; while at the same time the experiments upon the sheep's foot indicate that an ordinary solid has but a very limited range of operation upon the surrounding blood.f-, and that the clot which it induces does not propagate itself to more distant parts; so that the central portions of such a mass of blood should remain fluid, unless we admit that, when shed from the vessels, it is liberated from an influence which previously kept in check a spontaneous proneness to coagulation. Hence it seems likely that a foreign solid introduced into a vein acts not by creating a disposition to aggregate on the part of the fibrine, but by increasing a pre-existing tendency to it (as a thread induces the crystallization of sugar-candy), exalting the mutual attraction of its particles to a degree which overcomes a counteracting agency on the part of the tissues.

Further inquiry will, in all probability, throw clearer light upon this subject, but in the meantime the facts already known furnish to the unaided senses indisputable proof of the fundamental principle to which we were led by microscopical observation, viz. that the tissues through which the blood flows have, when healthy, special relations to the vital fluid, by virtue of which it is maintained in a fit state for transmission through the vessels. Further, the differences of adhesiveness in the corpuscles according as the blood is surrounded by healthy tissues or ordinary matter, can now be no longer matter of surprise, knowing as we do the alterations which take place in the chemical condition of the liquor sanguinis in consequence of such changes of circumstances, and also the great effect produced upon the adhesiveness of the red discs in blood outside the body by slight variations in the quality of the plasma.

The freedom from attraction for the fibrine, if not the actual repulsion of it, on the part of the walls of healthy blood-vessels, seems to explain the well-known fact in pathology, that when healthy capillaries are subjected to abnormal pressure in consequence of venous obstruction, the fluid squeezed through their parietes consists almost exclusively of serum; the fibrine being apparently excluded from their pores as liquid mercury is from those of flannel, or any other texture composed of a material destitute of attraction for it.

From the speedy coagulation of lymph effused into the interstices of inflamed organs or upon inflamed serous surfaces, compared with the length of time that blood has been known to remain fluid after being poured out into such situations in a state of health, and also from the deposition of fibrine which occurs at an early period upon the lining membrane of the vessels in arteritis or phlebitis, whether in the limited inflammation which results from the application of a ligature, or in the more extensive affection which is apt to occur spontaneously, it would appear that the liquor sanguinis, like the corpuscles, tends to comport itself near inflamed tissues as if in the vicinity of ordinary solid substances. It is true that coagulation is not observed to occur in the vessels of the frog's web after the application of irritants; but this is accounted for by the length of time required for the occurrence of the process within the vessels, the liquor sanguinis passing on into healthy regions, leaving the adhesive corpuscles behind it. Adhesiveness of corpuscles may, however, come on in circumstances which admit of permanent fluidity of the blood. Thus if a cat be killed without hemorrhage, and one of the jugular veins be exposed and tied in two places, and the animal be then suspended by the head so that the vein may be vertical in position, the upper part of the venous compartment included between the ligatures will within a very few minutes become colourless in consequence of rapid subsidence of the red corpuscles, implying that they are already closely aggregated, although, if the skin be carefully replaced so as to prevent drying of the tissues, the blood will remain fluid in that part of the vein for many hours. Whether the adhesiveness of the corpuscles in this case depend on a *post mortem* change in the vessels, or whether it is merely the result of the large size of the vein preventing the tissues from acting effectually on the blood, remains to be determined; but such a fact seems to prove that a higher grade of vital activity, so to speak, is required to prevent adhesiveness of corpuscles than to maintain the fluidity of the blood. Hence it is probable that, even if the blood were at rest in the vessels of a part, a stronger degree of irritation would be required in order to determine coagulation than would suffice to induce adhesiveness of the corpuscles, which seems to be a more sensitive test of a deviation of the tissues from the standard of health. I have however ascertained, by experiments upon the amputated sheep's foot, that if caustic ammonia is applied freely to a part of a vein after pressing the blood out of it, and the blood allowed to return when the ammoniacal odour has passed off, coagulation takes place in the portion of the vessel which has been so treated, although the chemical action of ammonia, if any of it remained in the tissues, would tend to prevent or check coagulation. I have also found a similar local clot form, though more slowly, after merely pinching a piece of a vein.

The principal results obtained in this section may be summed up as follows:-

The effects produced upon the circulation by the application of an irritant to a vascular part are twofold, consequent upon two primary changes in the tissues, which, though often concomitant, are entirely independent both in nature and mode of production. One of these is dilatation of the arteries (commonly preceded by a brief period of contraction), giving rise, in proportion to the increase of calibre, to more free flow through the capillaries, the blood remaining unaffected, except in the rate of its progress. This purely functional phenomenon is developed indirectly through the medium of the nervous system, being not limited to the part acted on by the irritant, but implicating a surrounding area of greater or less extent. The other change is the result of the direct operation of the irritating agent upon the tissues, which experience some alteration, in consequence of which the blood in their vicinity becomes impaired, losing the properties which characterise it while within a healthy part, and which render it fit for transmission through the vessels, and assuming those which it exhibits when removed from the body and placed in contact with ordinary solid matter. The first indication of this disorder of the vital fluid is, that its corpuscles, both red and white, acquire some degree of adhesiveness, which makes them prone to stick to one another and to the vascular parietes, and, lagging behind the liquor sanguinis, to accumulate in abnormal numbers in the minute vessels. This adhesiveness may exist, in proportion to the severity of the affection, in any degree, from that which merely gives rise to a very slight preponderance of the corpuscular elements of the blood in the part, up to that which induces complete obstruction of the capillaries; and when the irritation has been very severe, the liquor sanguinis also shows signs of participation in the lesion by a tendency to solidification of the fibrine.

SECTION IV: *On the Effects of Irritants upon the Tissues.*

The object of the present section is to inquire into the nature of that primary change which we have seen to be produced in the tissues by the direct action of irritants upon them.

The conclusion already arrived at, that blood flowing through an irritated part approaches more and more nearly, in proportion to the intensity of the affection, the condition which it assumes when separated from the living body, naturally leads us to infer that the tissues concerned are in some degree approximated to the state of ordinary matter, or, in other words, have suffered a diminution of power to discharge the offices peculiar to them as components of the healthy animal frame.

This inference is strongly supported by considering. What common effect is likely to be produced upon the tissues of the frog's web by all the various agents known to cause inflammatory congestion. To take first the case of mechanical violence. A forcible pinch of the delicate web seems likely, a priori, to impair its powers; for if the lesion be sufficiently severe, complete death of the part will result. An elevated temperature proves equally destructive if carried far enough; and its operation to a degree just short of this, while it produces congestion, can hardly fail to cause diminished vigour in the tissues. So also powerful chemical agents, if used cautiously, give rise to inflammation; but if otherwise, kill the part they act on. Even the pungent irritants which do not exert much chemical action, seem to benumb the energies of the spot to which they are applied. Thus a morsel of capsicum placed on the tip of the tongue speedily produces numbness there, and a piece of mustard lying on the finger for an hour or two dulls the sensibility of the skin. Chloroform, too, while it very readily induces stagnation followed by vesication in the frog's web, is an agent which appears likely to benumb the vital energies. If a small frog be put into a bottle of water highly charged with carbonic acid, and removed from it some time after all motion of the limbs has ceased, it will be found that, though the heart is still beating, the blood-vessels of the webs are loaded with stagnant corpuscles. After a while, however, resolution will take place, and some time later the animal will regain its consciousness. Here it appears probable that the carbonic acid, poisoning the web as well as the brain, paralyses for a time the functional activity of both; and that the return of the circulation, like the recovery of the cerebral functions, depends on a restoration of the dormant faculties of the affected tissues.

Perhaps the most instructive case is that of the galvanic shocli, which the following circumstances first showed mc to be capable of causing inflammatory congestion. Being desirous of ascertaining the effects of galvanism upon the cutaneous pigmentary system, I applied the poles of a battery in rather powerful action to the skin of the head of a frog, when, the shock affecting the brain, the animal was stunned and lay perfectly motionless. This state of things being favourable for pursuing my inquiry by aid of the microscope, I drew down one of the passive limbs, and having placed the foot under the instrument, arranged the fine platinum wire extremities of the poles at a short distance from one another at opposite sides of one of the webs, so that the current might pass through a part in the field of view, the circulation meanwhile remaining healthy. I now completed the circuit of the battery, when the leg became instantly drawn up by reflex action; yet on re-examination of the web, I found that, momentary as the shock had been, the part through which it had passed had become affected with intense inflammatory congestion, gradually shading off towards the healthy condition, which existed at a little distance. After about a quarter of an hour resolution of the confused mass of stagnant corpuscles occurred, and shortly after this the creature regained the power of voluntary motion. I afterwards repeated the experiment, both upon the same animal and upon another specimen, and always with the same results; and I particularly observed in one case that the white corpuscles were affected with great adhesiveness in the congested region.

With regard to the manner in which the abnormal condition of the blood was brought about in these cases, it has been already mentioned in Section I. that the galvanic current produces no increase of the adhesiveness of the red corpuscles of blood outside the body; but after what has been stated in the last Section, the reader will see no reason to think such an effect likely. It may, however, seem not improbable that the galvanic shock might, by its direct action upon the blood within the vessels, reduce it to the same condition as if removed from the body. But that this was not really the cause of the congestion, was clear from the fact that in the parts less intensely affected, where the corpuscles still moved slowly though possessed of considerable adhesiveness, the same condition continued long after all the blood which was in the vessels when the shock was transmitted had passed away. In this case therefore, as in all the others which we have considered, the blood was affected secondarily to the tissues. This being established, the natural interpretation of these experiments appears to be, that the portion of the web affected was, as it were, stunned by the shock, and its functions suspended like those of the brain; the resolution of the inflammation, like the return of volition, depending on recovery of function on the part of the tissues concerned.

From such considerations as these, it appears that all those agents which produce inflammatory congestion when applied to the web, though differing widely in their nature, agree in having a tendency to inflict lesion upon the tissues and impair their functional activity.

But powerful as are the arguments thus obtained by inference, it is very desirable to confirm them by direct observation, and it fortunately happens that the cutaneous pigmentary system of the frog is a tissue which discharges functions very apparent to the eye, so that it is easy to trace their modifications under the influence of irritation.

In the first experiment with mustard described in the last section (performed September 29th, 1856), the space on which the irritant had acted presented a very striking difference from the rest of the web in the appearance of the pigment, which in healthy parts was in the form of small roundish black dots; while in the mustard area, and accurately corresponding to the extent of stagnation in the capillaries, each spot was extended to a stellate figure.

I thus became for the first time aware that the pigment is capable of variations, and my attention having been directed to the subject, I soon found that similar changes occur spontaneously, and give rise to alterations in the colour of the skin, which is paler in proportion as the colouring matter is more completely collected into round spots. For some weeks I supposed myself to have been the first discoverer of this curious fact, till I was referred by Dr. SHARPEY to the recent labours of the Germans on the subject. They, however, as I afterwards found, had taken an entirely erroneous view of the phenomenon, attributing the round form of the masses of pigment to contraction of the branching offsets of stellate cells; whereas it turned out that the chromatophorous cells do not alter in form, but that the colourless fluid and dark molecules which constitute their contents are capable of remarkable variations in relative distribution, the molecules being sometimes all congregated in the central parts of the cells, the offsets containing merely invisible fluid, while at other times the colouring particles are diffused throughout their complicated and delicate branches; and between these extremes any intermediate condition may be assumed. It further appeared that concentration of pigment takes place in obedience to nervous influence, while diffusion, though also an active vital process, tends to occur when the pigment-cells are liberated from the action of the nerves. But for further particulars on this subject,

I beg to refer the reader to the immediately preceding paper in this volume.

The contrast between the pigment in the area on which the mustard had acted and that of surrounding parts in the case last alluded to, at once strucli me as probably the result of a direct action exercised upon the tissues by the irritant. It seemed possible, however, that it might be a secondary effect of the state of the blood in the congested vessels; and in order to ascertain which was the truth, I performed, on the 14th of October, the following experiment:

Having cut out a piece of the web of a healthy frog, I placed a small portion of mustard upon its centre when all the blood had escaped from it. After a while the spots of pigment seen through the thin margin of the mustard, presented a stellate form, while in the rest of the piece they were still of a rounded figure. Hence it was clear that the change in the disposition of the pigment was the result of the direct action of the mustard upon the tissues of the web.

A new field of investigation was thus opened before me, promising to throw great light upon the nature of inflammation.

To explain the effects of irritants upon the pigmentary tissue proved, however, to be a matter of considerable difficulty. Tincture of cantharides and croton oil, which happened to be among the first substances which I employed with reference to this subject, resembled mustard in causing diffusion of the pigment. Taking, in the first instance, the same view of this change as the German authorities, I attributed it to the relaxation of contractile cells, and regarded its occurrence, in consequence of irritation, as an indication of loss of power in the tissues, a view which was in harmony with the nature of the derangement of th; blood in a congested part. Crotan oil, curiously enough, acted verv slowly on the web, not producing any change on either pigment or blood for an hour or more: also its effects appeared inconsistent with my theory; for while it ultimately gave rise to diffusion of the pigment to even a greater extent than I had seen occur with mustard, yet it induced only comparatively slight appearances of congestion. Chloroform also seemed at first still more anomalous in its operation, though in the opposite way; for though it was pre-eminently potent in inducing congestion, it caused no alteration whatever in the appearance of the pigment, whether mildly or strongly applied.

Afterwards, as the true nature of the pigmentary functions became unveiled, and further facts were developed, these difficulties were completely cleared away. The first step towards their solution was made in an experiment with ammonia. A frog being placed under chloroform, I covered the whole of the foot with sweet oil, except a small area in one of the webs, the pigment being in the stellate condition, i.e. about midway between perfect concentration and full diffusion. An assistant then held at a short distance above it a piece of lint soaked in the strongest liquor ammonia, so that its pungent alkaline vapour might play upon the exposed area, while the rest of the foot was protected by the oil. This having been continued for a few seconds, accumulation of corpuscles and stagnation occurred in the vessels of the area, without any change in the appearance of the pigment. After a while, however, the creature happened to grow pale, and, in the web generally, the pigment became completely concentrated so as to assume the dotted aspect, but in the part which was the seat of congestion it remained stellate as before. Hence it appeared that though the ammonia did not cause any change in the distribution of the pigment, it had in reality produced a great effect upon the chromatophorous cells, which, in the area exposed to its influence, had been deprived of the power of concentration by the mildest degree of action of the alkali that sufficed to induce stagnation of the blood. 011 examination of the web about four hours later, resolution of the stagnation was found to have taken place, though there was still some excess of corpuscles, with marked adhesiveness of the colourless ones in the vessels of the ammonia area. The creature was now released for the night. Next morning the integument was in the opposite extreme of colour, being almost black, and the pigment had the reticular appearance, being fully diffused throughout the whole web, except the central part of the ammonia area, where it retained the same stellate condition as the day before. Hence it appeared probable that the diffusive power, as well as the concentrating, had been paralysed by the ammonia, but had been recovered in all the area except the part that was likely to be the last to regain its functions. To ascertain whether the concentrating power had also been regained, I killed the frog and amputated the leg; soon after which the usual *post mortem* concentration took place completely in the web generally, while in the central part of the area the medium state was still retained, and in the rest of its extent concentration considerably beyond the medium state, but short of the full degree, supervened, showing that recovery of function had taken place to a considerable extent, but was not yet quite complete.

I now felt little doubt that chloroform also possessed the power of arresting the pigmentary functions; but in order to prove the fact I killed a dark frog, and placed one of its legs in that fluid for half a minute, and then wrapped both it and the other leg in damp lint. After some hours the limb which had not been treated with chloroform was quite pale, while the other, having lost the faculty of *post mortem* concentration, remained as dark as before. The appearance presented by the pigment in the two feet is shown in Plate XLVII. figs. 1 and 2.

Mechanical violence proved similar in its effects on the pigment, which, in the area pinched, retained the same appearance as before, except that in parts where the pressure operated most severely the cells seemed sometimes to have suffered rupture, Fig. 2, Plate XLVIII, is a camera lucida sketch of part of a spot which had been compressed by means of padded forceps, with an adjoining uninjured portion of the web. The pigment was fully diffused before the experiment was performed, and remained so afterwards in the area squeezed, while it became concentrated elsewhere, and this was the condition of things when the drawing was made. The concomitant differences in tint between the blood in the affected and the sound parts in consequence of the accumulation of closely packed red discs in the former, are also strikingly shown in the sketch.

The galvanic shock, too, produced no effect apparent to the eye upon the pigment of the parts in which it caused stagnation of the blood, but experiments afterwards made showed me that, like ammonia, it exerted a paralysing agency both upon the concentrating and the diffusive powers; and the same results ensued 011 the application of dry heat in the cases mentioned in the last section.

From these and other similar facts it appeared that mustard, croton oil, and cantharides are exceptional as regards the diffusion to which they give rise, the usual course being that irritants, when applied so as to produce stagnation of the blood, suspend at the same time both the functions of the pigment-cells.

It afterwards turned out that mustard was, in reality, no exception to this general rule. Subsequent experiments showed that diffusion takes place to very different degrees in different instances under the action of this substance, but that in all cases, after reaching a certain point, it becomes incapable of advancing further in the irritated part, however much it may increase in the body generally, in case of the animal changing to a darker colour. These differences depend partly upon the strength of the mustard, the diffusion being least when the irritant is most potent. Thus, on one occasion, when a solution of the volatile oil in spirit of wine was applied to a web in which the pigment was fully concentrated, congestion was very rapidly developed, without any alteration in the appearance of the chromatophorous cells. That the diffusion is in inverse proportion to the energy with which the mustard acts, was well illustrated by the experiment which furnished the drawing given in Plate XLVIII. fig. 1. In that case, a frog having been prepared in the manner mentioned in the note to page 611, a portion of very strong mustard was placed upon the middle of one of the webs, the pigment being in the stellate condition, such as is seen on the left-hand side of the sketch, which represents a part of the edge of the spot to which the irritant was applied, together with an adjoining portion of the web. Shortly after this had been done, I noticed that the pigment was in a state of full diffusion in a ring round about the opaque mass, producing the reticular appearance shown in the stripe down the middle of the sketch. I had in a previous case seen a similar ring become affected with congestion, when a portion of mustard had been applied for a long time, in consequence of the pungent vapour of the volatile oil playing upon the neighbouring parts of the web, and there could be no doubt that the effect on the pigment in the present instance was due to the same cause; but in the latter no material change was as yet visible in the blood except close to the edge of the mustard, where the corpuscles were seen to be abnormally adhesive.

After the lapse of about an hour, the area on which the irritant had lain being examined, was found to be the seat of the most intense inflammatorycongestion, indicated in the drawing by the crimson colour of the vessels, but the pigment there had experienced only an exceedingly slight degree of diffusion, being, in fact, almost exactly in the same state as at the commencement of the experiment. Thus the vapour of the volatile oil, though operating too mildly to cause inflammatory congestion, nevertheless induced the highest possible degree of pigmentary diffusion; but the mustard, where it lay actually in contact with the web, and acted energetically upon it, arrested that very process of diffusion to which its gentler operation gives rise.

In the progress of the case it happened that the animal changed from the medium tint which it had at first to a very pale colour, the pigment, in the web generally, assuming the dotted condition depicted on the right-hand side of the drawing. Yet many hours after the mustard had been removed, the pigment on which it had acted retained its stellate disposition, and the reticular appearance in the surrounding ring also remained unchanged, showing that the power of concentration had been permanently lost in those parts, and affording a favourable opportunity for obtaining by means of the camera lucida a delineation of the medium, and both extreme conditions of the pigment in the same web. Next day the experiment was rendered still more instructive by the skin becoming excessively dark, the pigment undergoing full diffusion in the healthy parts of the web, so that the contrast between the ring about the congested area and the surrounding regions no longer existed: yet the stellate condition was still maintained where the mustard had lain, showing that it had suspended the faculty of diffusion no less than that of concentration.

Croton oil now no longer seemed anomalous in its operation. Its curiously slow action upon the frog is comparable to the mild influence of the vapour of mustard, and the slight amount of inflammatory appearance which I had sometimes observed in a part where it had caused a great degree of pigmentary diffusion, is strictly analogous to the healthy state of the circulation in the reticular ring round the congested area in the last experiment.

Cantharides also presents a parallel case. Its action is even more slow than that of croton oil; and on referring to notes taken at an early period in this investigation, I find that in one instance, when two hours and a half had elapsed after the application of a small drop of the tincture to the web, though diffusion of the pigment had become apparent in the area on which it had acted, no change of the blood had yet been observed; and an hour and a half later, the red corpuscles, though abnormally adhesive as compared with those in surrounding parts of the web, were still moving slowly through the vessels.

Hence it appears that diffusion of the pigment may be produced by either of these three substances without the blood undergoing any material derangement, and therefore that its occurrence under their influence is to a great extent, if not entirely, independent of the inflammatory process. On the other hand, it has been demonstrated, as regards mustard, that when stagnation of the blood has been developed through its action, the state of the pigment-cells is the same as is induced by irritants generally, viz. a complete suspension of functional activity; and, from analogy, we may be pretty sure that this is also true of croton oil and cantharides, although their slow operation renders it difficult to obtain absolute proof upon the point.

In a physiological point of view, it is an interesting question, what is the cause of the diffusion of the pigment induced by these three irritants. I have shown elsewhere that concentration is the invariable result of the action of the nerves upon the chromatophorous cells, and that diffusion takes place whenever they are liberated from nervous influence. Also in the tree-frog of the Continent, which is much more liable to changes in the colour of the integument, in consequence of direct irritation, than our own species, the invariable experience of the German observers was, that concentration followed the application of a local stimulus, while secondary diffusion sometimes occurred in the irritated spot, depending apparently upon exhaustion From these facts, diffusion ensuing on irritation cannot well be regarded as an increased action excited by the stimulus, but rather as an evidence of diminished vigour. With croton oil and cantharides, which have not an irritating vapour, the diffusion is exactly limited to the extent of the irritant, showing that it is due to a direct action on the tissues; and the most probable explanation of its occurrence appears to be that mustard, croton oil, and cantharides have the peculiarity among irritants of affecting the nerves of the pigment-cells in the part they act on, somewhat more rapidly than the cells themselves, and, paralysing the former while the latter still retain their powers more or less intact, permit diffusion to go on unrestrained by nervous influence, till the further operation of the irritant completely suspends the pigmentary functions. It may be objected to this view, that diffusion occurs on the application of these substances to an amputated limb, but, from evidence given elsewhere, it is probable that the pigment cells possess a local nervous apparatus, on which the occurrence and maintenance of post mortem concentration depend, and the paralysis of which, while the pigment-cells retain their powers, would give rise to diffusion in an amputated limb. Be this as it may, the fact that the state of full diffusion continued in the ring around the congested area in the last mustard experiment for hours after the irritant had been removed, although, during that time, complete concentration occurred in the web generally, is pretty clear evidence that the pigment-cells in that part had not merely been stimulated to increased action (for in that case they would have returned to their former condition soon after the stimulus had ceased to operate), but had suffered a loss of the faculty of concentration. Whether the loss of power resided in the nerves of the pigment-cells, or in those cells themselves, is a matter of indifference as regards the objects of the present inquiry; the important fact being that an action of the mustard so mild as to give rise to little or no derangement of the blood, nevertheless produced a certain degree of loss of power in the part on which it operated. There can be no doubt that the same principles apply to the cases of croton oil and cantharides; and thus the diffusion caused by these three irritants assumes a high interest, as visible evidence of diminished functional activity accompanying, if not preceding, the earliest approaches to inflammatory congestion in parts which have been subjected to their influence.

With the view of ascertaining the nature of the effect produced on the pigment-cells by the mildest action of chloroform which is capable of causing inflammatory disorder, I ascertained, by repeated experiments, the shortest time in which the vapour of that liquid gave rise to unequivocal signs of a congestive tendency in the web of the living frog; and having found this to be about half a minute, suspended one of the legs of a recently killed dark frog in a vessel, the bottom of which was covered with chloroform, having previously examined the webs microscopically, and found that full diffusion of pigment existed throughout them. The result was that the limb exposed to the chloroform vapour remained dark, while the other became gradually pale. On re-examination of the former after some hours, each web presented stripes of full diffusion of pigment alternating with others in a medium condition; their direction being at right angles to the margin of the web. The longitudinal folds in which the webs had happened to be, had prevented the chloroform vapour from gaining equally free access to all parts; yet the chromatophorous cells in the stripes that had been thus partially protected from its influence had been incapable of complete concentration, showing that even the exceedingly slight degree of action which the chloroform could have exerted upon these places sufficed to diminish, though not to destroy, the functional activity: of the pigmentary tissue.

In one of the experiments performed in order to determine the effect of mechanical violence, as before alluded to, the pigment remained unchanged for days in the area which had been pinched, while varying in other parts of the web; yet, though great excess of red corpuscles existed in the vessels of the affected spot, they never ceased to move; showing that the functions of the pigment-cells might be completely suspended by a degree of irritation short of that which occasions actual stagnation of the blood.

The same thing was afterwards seen in a case in which a small drop of wood-vinegar was placed upon one of the webs of a frog which had been deprived of the power of voluntarily moving the limbs by passing a knife between the occiput and the atlas, so as to sever the brain from the cord. The fluid being thus allowed to lie quite undisturbed, did not spread at all upon the web, which was dry before it was applied. It produced its effects very slowly, so that, after the lapse of three and a half hours, the blood in the area covered by it, while everywhere presenting inflammatory appearances, was still only partially stagnant. Yet throughout this space the, pigment retained exactly the same moderate degree of diffusion as it had at the beginning of the experiment, although in the interval complete concentration had taken place elsewhere; and a very striking contrast was presented between the stellate pigment with the adhesive though still moving blood-corpuscles where the web was wet with the vinegar, and the dotted pigment and perfectly healthy circulation in the dry parts immediately adjacent.

Seeing, then, that complete suspension of the pigmentary functions may be caused by an amount of irritation which induces only a minor degree of congestion, and further, that (as we learn from the experiment with chloroform vapour) a still milder operation of an irritant renders these functions sluggish though not completely arresting them, we seem to have sufficient evidence that impairment of the functional activity of the chroinatophorous cells occurs in the very earliest stages of that primary change in the tissues which leads to inflammatory derangement of the blood.

It was seen in the ammonia experiment related above, that resolution having taken place in the congested area, the pigment-cells of the part recovered the faculty both of diffusion and concentration. This might have been pretty confidently predicted; for as congestion is a necessary consequence of the disorder produced in the tissues by irritants, we might have been almost sure that the return of the vital fluid to that healthy condition in which it is fit for free transmission through the vessels, must be preceded by a restoration of the living solids to their normal state. In the case alluded to, however, no sign of recovery of the pigment-cells appeared till after the circulation had become re-established; and even when several hours had elapsed, they still remained paralysed in the central part of the area on which the ammonia had acted. This is in harmony with the fact lately pointed out, that complete suspension of the pigmentary functions may accompany a state of the blood short of actual stagnation; and both appear to depend upon the circumstance that the chromatophorous cells are an extremely delicate form of tissue.

The rate of recovery of the pigment-cells varies greatly, however, in different cases, and in this respect much depends upon the nature of the irritant. An example of an agent of this class producing only very transient effects on the pigmentary functions is presented by carbonic acid. It has been before mentioned that the immersion of a living frog for about a quarter of an hour in water highly charged with that gas, gives rise to complete stagnation of the blood in the webs, although the heart still continues beating, but. that resolution occurs after the animal has been exposed for awhile to the atmosphere. With a view to ascertaining whether the congestion was due to the direct action of the acid upon the tissues, I made the following experiment. Having killed a dark frog and amputated both legs, and ascertained by microscopic examination that the pigment was fully diffused in the webs, I put one limb into a bottle of aerated water and the other into ordinary water: the latter soon became pale through post mortem concentration, but the former remained as dark as ever during the two hours for which it was retained in the solution of carbonic acid, the direct action of which upon the bloodless tissues was thus demonstrated. An hour after the limb had been taken out, however, it was evidently recovering, being distinctly lighter in colour than it had been, and two hours later it was quite pale, and the pigment in the webs was found to be in almost the extreme degree of concentration. In subsequent similar experiments I left the leg in the aerated water for a longer time, during which it always retained precisely the same tint that it had when first introduced; and, if left for many hours, showed signs of loss of vitality, by the early supervention of cadaveric rigidity and exfoliation of the epidermis; but if it was taken out within about four hours, the pigment-cells recovered completely; and in one case a leg not removed for nine hours regained, nevertheless, to a considerable extent, the faculty of concentration. Thus it appears that carbonic acid, though exercising a powerful sedative influence upon the tissues, and paralysing for the time their vital energies, so as to give rise to intense inflammatory congestion, yet, even after a very protracted action, leaves them in a state susceptible of speedy recovery.

Here we see for the first time a satisfactory solution of the much-debated problem of the cause of congestion of the lungs in Asphyxia; for there can, I conceive, be no doubt that the pulmonary tissues, exposed under ordinary circumstances to the influence of a free supply of oxygen, suffer, like those of the frog's web, from the vicinity of an abnormal proportion of carbonic acid, and inflammatory congestion is the necessary consequence. At the same time, the rapid recovery of the lungs from asphyxial congestion of considerable duration, when the normal atmosphere is readmitted, finds an equally close parallel in the speedy return both of the pigment-cells and the blood to the healthy condition when the foot of the frog is removed from the aerated water.

But the most important lesson to be learnt from these simple experiments with carbonic acid upon amputated limbs, is that the tissues possess, independently of the central organs of the nervous system, or of the circulation, or even of the presence of blood within the vessels, an intrinsic power of recovery from irritation, when it has not been carried beyond a certain point; a principle of fundamental importance, which has never before, so far as I am aware, been established or conjectured. It applies equally in the case of other irritants. Thus having transmitted for about a quarter of a minute, through one of the webs of a dark amputated limb, powerful galvanic currents, such as I had before ascertained to cause stagnation of the blood when operating for an instant upon the living animal, I found, after the lapse of an hour and a quarter, that the process of concentration had advanced considerably in the next web, but in that on which the galvanism had acted had only just commenced, even in the parts most remote from the point to which the poles of the battery were applied; while in the vicinity of that spot the state of full diffusion still continued. After the lapse of three more hours, however, the pigment was almost fully concentrated in the part of the web where it was before only slightly so; and even where it had been most directly subjected to the galvanic influence, it had undergone a certain, though very slight degree of the same change, the chromatophorous cells having even there partially recovered their functions.

This inherent power in the tissues of recovering from the effects of irritation, explains the occurrence of resolution in an amputated limb, such as I once observed in a case where a moderate amount of congestion had been induced under the action of oil of turpentine before the animal was killed, and the blood resumed to a great extent its normal characters in the vessels several hours after the limb had been severed from the body.

The return of the blood along with the tissues to the state of health is a very interesting circumstance. Whether it depends upon an intrinsic power of recovery on the part of the vital fluid, or on the living solids resuming an active operation upon it, is at present uncertain; but in the mean time, the phenomena of resolution already assume a far more intelligible aspect than heretofore, on the hypothesis that the tissues generally are endowed with the same faculty of self-restoration as the pigment-cells.

It may be well to give here a list of all the agents whose effects upon the pigmentary functions I have investigated. They are as follows: Mechanical violence, the galvanic shock, desiccation of the tissues, dry heat, warm water at 100' Fahrenheit, intense cold, caustic ammonia, a strong solution of common salt, carbonic acid, acetic acid, tincture of iodine, chloroform, oil of turpentine, mustard, tincture of cantharides, and croton oil. These are all of them irritants, ie. give rise to inflammatory congestion through their direct action upon a vascular part, as I have witnessed in the frog's web in every case except that of cold, the influence of which in causing intense inflammation in the human subject is, however, familiar to all. All of them also afforded, in their effects upon the pigment-cells, ocular evidence of impairment of the functional activity of the tissues on which they act; and considering the number included in the list, and their great variety in essential nature, we need not hesitate to admit that similar effects are produced by the entire class of irritants.

There is another tissue in the frog's web which discharges functions apparent to the eye, viz. the arterial muscular fibre-cells, the contractions of which are readily recognized in consequence of the changes of calibre which they produce in the vessels; and the manner in which the arteries are affected in a congested part of the web indicates that the muscular, like the pigmentary tissue, has its functional activity impaired by a certain amount of irritation. Thus I have repeatedly been struck with the fact, and noted it before I knew its significance, that an artery running through a limited area on which an irritant has acted, remains dilated in the spot, although it may vary in other parts of its course. This I have observed in one experiment with mustard, in one with acetic acid, in two with ammonia, and in one with heat. In the last-mentioned case the appearance was particularly striking, from the circumstance that two arteries happened to pass through the burnt part, and were constricted to absolute closure in the rest of their course, contrasting strongly with their fully dilated state within the area.

In the ammonia experiments also the artery concerned was, in the progress of each case, seen to be completely constricted beyond the congested area, though still dilated within it. The limitation of this effect on the arteries, to the extent of the part acted un by the irritant, proves that it is the result of its direct action on the tissues; differing remarkably in this respect from the dilatation of the vessels, which is produced indirectly through the medium of the nervous system, and affects a wide space round about the spot irritated,

But with regard to both the muscular fibre-cells of the arteries and the pigment-cells, it may fairly be questioned whether the diminution of power to act resides in them or in those portions of their nerves which are situated in the irritated region. The view that the nerves are paralysed by irritants is consistent with the benumbing influence well known to be exerted upon the human skin or mucous membranes by some of those agents, e.g., mechanical violence, the galvanic shock, cold, and chloroform. I have also observed, as before alluded to, that mustard produces a similar result on the cutaneous sensory nerves, and hence it seems probable that the same is true of the whole class of irritants. Again, the diffusion induced by mustard, croton oil, and cantharides indicates, according to what we have seen to be its most probable explanation, that the nerves of the pigment-cells suffer impairment of functional activity under the action of these three substances. On the other hand, the fact that diffusion is arrested equally with concentration by most irritants, appears to prove that the chromatophorous cell8 are themselves also affected with loss of power; for, as has been before alluded to, the withdrawal of nervous influence from them in a healthy state of the tissues invariably gives rise to diffusion, and the same result would necessarily follow the action of an irritant which merely paralysed the nerves. I have also observed, on two occasions, after the energetic operation of an irritant upon a part of a web containing a large artery, that drawing the point of a needle firmly across the vessel failed to induce the slightest contraction in it, even at the very point crossed by the needle; proving that the muscular fibre-cells had lost their irritability. At the same time it is by no means improbable that the nerves of the arteries may suffer before their muscular constituents, just as in the intestines, after death, the functions of the intrinsic nervous apparatus are lost some time before muscular contractility ceases.

The question whether the suspension of function induced by irritants is conked to the nerves or affects the tissues generally, being one of great interest, I was anxious to obtain clear evidence regarding it; and it occurred to me that valuable information would probably be derived from observing the effects of such agents upon the action of the cilia, which, though not present in the web of the frog, exist in abundance upon the mucous surfaces of the mouth and cesophagus of that animal. Dr. SHARPEY in his celebrated article "Cilia" in the "Enyclopedia of Anatomy and Physiology,' mentions experiments made by PURKINJE and VALENTIN, and also by himself, with a great variety of substances, including among the rest some irritants, which, when applied with sufficient energy, arrested completely, by their chemical action as it was supposed, the movements of the lashing filaments. It is evident, however, that in order to produce effects at all comparable to the state of the tissues of the frog's web in congestion, it would be necessary to adopt some more delicate method of experimenting, and the most eligible means for this purpose seemed to be to allow an irritating vapour to play upon a ciliated surface. Accordingly, on the 30th of November, 1857+, having cut off a small piece of the tongue of a frog killed about an hour before, and placed it upon a slip of glass under the microscope, with just enough water to permit the free play of the cilia, I held near to it a piece of lint soaked in chloroform, keeping my eye over the microscope. The effect was instantaneous cessation of the previously rapid action of the cilia, which now stood out straight and motionless, like the hairs of a brush. I now immediately withdrew the lint, after which the same state of complete inaction continued for about half a minute, when languid movements began to show themselves, and after the lapse of five minutes more the ciliary action was going on pretty briskly in some parts, and ten minutes later seemed to have almost completely recovered.

Thus chloroform vapour produced in the ciliated epithelium-cells a condition precisely similar to that brought about in the pigment-cells by irritants applied so as to cause inflammatory congestion of the web, viz. a state of suspension or temporary deprivation of functional activity. And as the removal of the epithelium-cells from the surface on which they grow does not arrest the movements of their cilia, no mere paralysis of nerves could account for this result, which necessarily implied that the epithelial tissue itself was affected with loss of power to discharge its accustomed functions. In repetitions of this procedure upon the same and other portions of the tongue, I did not generally get complete cessation of movement of all the cilia, but usually some retained a languid action, which improved after the chloroform had been removed. In one instance, however, the same perfect stoppage took place as in the first case, and the recovery was also very general, though the returning action was languid. Under these circumstances, a piece of lint dipped in strongest liquor ammoniae was brought within about 1½ inch of the object, and retained there for about fifty seconds, during which time the ciliary motion became progressively and greatly diminished, and within twenty-five seconds of the removal of the lint, had ceased altogether. Some water was then added, so as to get rid of the absorbed alkali, when the cilia soon began to move again, and within about three minutes their play was more vigorous and general than before the ammonia was used, and three minutes later it was universal, as it was prior to the application of the chloroform. On another occasion, in a different animal, the cilia having been ascertained to be in rapid motion on a fresh piece of tongue, lint containing liquor ammoniae was held at a short distance from it for thirty-three seconds. The cilia very soon grew languid, and by the end of the time mentioned had quite ceased to act. The lint was at once withdrawn, but no recovery occurred; the operation of the irritant had been rather too energetic, and the vitality of the tissue had been destroyed. A languid state of the cilia was also produced by placing freshly prepared mustard near them, and improvement took place when it had been removed; but the essential oil itself, applied on lint like the chloroform and ammonia, though not acting so rapidly as might have been expected, permanently arrested the vibratile filaments. The vapour of strong acetic acid, if acting for four seconds, caused great diminution of the motion, and in another instance arrested it completely in five seconds. I did not, however, see any recovery from the effects of this agent, which produced obvious organic injury in the cells. The introduction of a portion of the mucous membrane of the mouth into a bottle of aerated water for about twenty minutes gave rise to permanent stoppage of the cilia, and similar treatment for three or four hours caused disorganization of the epithelium, whereas the same period of immersion in ordinary water did not arrest the cilia. Powerful interrupted galvanic currents, transmitted for a few seconds through a particular spot in a piece of tongue on which the cilia were in free movement, abraded a portion of the epithelium there, and arrested completely the cilia of adjacent cells still *in situ.* and rendered those of other parts of the specimen extremely languid in their action. But the most satisfactory results were obtained from experiments with heat, which has the great advantage over chemical irritants, that it leaves no material behind it to act upon the delicate tissue. On the 14th of December, 1857, having ascertained that steeping a piece of the tongue of a frog for five minutes in water of 110' Fahrenheit used total and permanent cessation of ciliary action and desquamation of the epithelium, at 9h 9m P.M. I placed a portion of that organ, in which the vibratile movements were equable though rather languid, in water at 100' FAHR and retained it there for a minute and a quarter, when it was transferred to cold water. On examining it after the lapse of nearly two minutes, I found the cilia acting decidedly more briskly than at first, but in the course of the next quarter of an hour they flagged very much, and in many parts ceased to move altogether. By this time I had fixed the specimen securely at the bottom of a glass trough, which I now suddenly filled up with water at 102' FAHR and on first catching sight of the object, within a quarter of a minute of this procedure, found all the cilia absolutely motionless. I then at once drew off the warm water with a siphon previously arranged; and no sooner had this been done, than movements already began to show themselves in the cilia, and their action increased rapidly on my filling up the trough with cold water, and in a short time was all but universal and brisk, far superior to what it was before the hot water was put in. After a few minutes more, however, it was again very languid, and ceased entirely in many parts. I now, at 9h 38m, filled up the trough with water at 104' FAHR. at 9h 38m the cilia were almost all motionless; by 9h 38m 55s the trough had been again emptied, but at 9h 39m 5s there was even less movement seen. Cold water was again poured in at 9h 39m 35s, and after eighteen seconds, action was reappearing in the cilia, and it continued to increase during the next seven minutes, at the end of which time it was again almost universal. At 9h 52m the cold water was drawn off, and the same condition of the cilia having been ascertained to exist, the trough was, at 9h 53m 27s, filled up again with water at 104' FAHR;. Eighteen seconds after this had been done, the ciliary action was found much diminished, but had not fully ceased; and after nine seconds more, during which the warm water was drawn off, the cilia were still acting very slightly. Within twenty-three seconds of this time the trough was again filled with cold water: now, however, the epithelium was in many parts beginning to exfoliate, swelling up by endosmose in obedience to the ordinary laws of chemical affinity, and so indicating that it was losing its vitality. I also lost sight of the precise spot which I had been observing, but noticed that ciliary action was again going on pretty quickly in some places. There can be no doubt, although there was no opportunity for observing the fact, that the first immersion in hot water caused cessation of the ciliary action; and that being admitted, we have in this case suspension of function and recovery four times repeated in the same fragment of tissue in consequence of as many applications and withdrawals of the irritant. It is a curious circumstance that each recovery, except the final one, brought up the action of the cilia for a time to a better state than they had just before the last introduction of warm water. But the discussion of this and other circumstances in this case will be best reserved till after the mention of another set of experiments.

In order to eliminate the nerves completely from among the causes both of the suspension of function produced by irritants and the recovery from that state, it seemed desirable, if possible, to observe those occurrences in detached epithelium-cells, and on the 22nd of January 1859 I made the attempt to do so. At first, however, it proved more difficult than I had anticipated. It was of course easy to obtain the material to operate on, by gently scraping the surface of the palate of a recently killed frog with a knife, and placing the mucus-like product on a plate of glass with a drop of water. But the tissue thus separated from its connections was in an exceedingly delicate condition, and any agent used for arresting the action of the cilia was very apt to destroy at the same time the vitality of the cells. Thus when the object was warmed by placing the glass plate on a piece of iron at about 100' FAHR for half a minute, the vibratory movements were arrested, but never recovered, and in a short time the cells swelled up by endosmose. It appeared probable that the tissue had suffered during the time required for the cooling of the glass; and in order to avoid this, and also prevent the object-glass becoming obscured by vapour from the warm water condensing upon it, the epithelium was placed between two slips of thin covering glass, kept from too close approximation by fragments of the same material interposed, the whole forming a layer so thin that it would be rapidly heated if any hot body were placed in its vicinity, and cool as quickly on its removal. A small cautery iron, with a bulbous extremity about as big as a hazelnut, just too hot to bear in contact with the finger, was now put behind the stage of the microscope, within about three-quarters of an inch of the object, the diaphragm plate having been removed to afford room for this being done without interfering with the light sent up by the reflector. The result, which I watched from the first, was the same that f had once before observed from the very gentle application of heat to a portion of a frog's tongue, viz. primary increase in the action of the cilia which had previously been languid, but which, within ten seconds of the approxima- tion of the cautery, were moving with great rapidity, and con- tinued to do so for about twenty-five seconds, at the expiration of which their motion was seen to be diminishing, and after another minute and a half it was considerably more languid than at the beginning of the experiment. The cautery being now removed was found to be much cooled though still warm, and its withdrawal did not affect the cilia, which still remained much in the same state after the lapse of eight minutes. I now repeated the experiment upon a fresh portion of epithelium, but this time used the cautery red-hot, placing it about 2 inches behind the object: no sooner had this been done than the action of the cilia became excessively increased, but this did not continue for more than five seconds, when they became perfectly motionless. The hot iron was now at once withdrawn, but the cilia under spe- cial observation did not recover. In other situations in the same specimen, however, movements were observed in the course of the following minute, and it was still continuing seven minutes later, when a part having been brought into the field where there were two considerable groups of cells in moderate activity, the cautery was again applied at a distance of about 24 inches. The motions of the cilia immediately became distinctly increased, but, as in the former case, this condition gave place in five seconds to universal quiescence. The iron was then removed, and on re-examination after three minutes, the cilia were again moving, though in a somewhat languid manner in both parts of the field. For the sake of confirmation I again operated in a similar manner upon another specimen, on which I performed no less than five successive experiments with similar results in all. In the first three of these trials I had the very same cilia under observation, and saw them time after time become first increased in action and then arrested under the influence of the cautery, and gradually recover after its removal. In some instances the times of cessation and of recovery were noted as follows:- In the first the cilia were arrested in two seconds after the application of the hot iron, but the exact time of recovery was not observed; in the second, cessation of movement was produced in two seconds, and return began in fifteen seconds; in the third, cessation was fifteen seconds, and recovery also in fifteen seconds; in the fourth, the times were not noted; in the fifth, movement ceased in about two seconds and returned in twenty. The experiments were performed within about five minutes of each other, or sometimes less. It is also to be remarked, that there were some slight differences in the degree of heat of the cautery and its vicinity to the object.

These experiments are as instructive as they are simple and easy of performance. They show conclusively that a component tissue of the animal frame may, independently of the nervous system, have its actions either excited or paralysed by the direct operation of an irritant upon it, and that it may possess an equally independent power of recovery. Also in the accelerated movements of the cilia elicited by very gentle heat, as compared with the cessation of their vibrations under a higher temperature, we have a striking confirmation of the view which I had taken of the relaxation of the arteries and hollow viscera in consequence of nervous irritation. For the law which we thus see regulating the effects of heat upon the epithelium-cells is precisely that which I had inferred must govern the action of afferent nerves upon nerve-cells; this law being, that an agency which, when operating mildly, stimulates a tissue to increased activity, may, when more energetic, temporarily arrest its functions. Whether or not the converse always holds, viz, that any agent which is capable of suspending the functional activity of a tissue may also excite it if applied with sufficient gentleness, or, in other words, whether irritants are in all cases also stimulants, seems very doubtful. As regards the nerves, such does appear to be the case; for while many, and probably all influences which induce inflammatory congestion cause temporary paralysis of sensation in parts on which they act severely enough, they all stimulate the afferent nerves in the first instance, as is shown by the reflex changes in the calibre of the arteries which occur round about any irritated spot. The nervous centres, too, present an illustration of the same principle, not only in the effects produced upon them by the nerves, as lately alluded to, but also in the excitement well known to be occasioned by small doses of many sedative narcotics, such as alcohol, opium, and chloroform, which may be regarded as special irritants of the nervous centres. In the case of the cilia, I have not observed primary increase of movement to be induced by any agent besides heat; but I am not prepared to say that it might not by careful management be made to occur with some other irritants.

The pigment-cells in the common frog give very little indication of the stimulating properties of irritants, as is evident from several of the experiments which have been recorded in this section. In the tree frog, however, as we are informed by the German authorities, a part of the integument subjected to such influences rapidly assumes a pale tint, and that even in a portion of skin removed from the body. I have also several times noticed, after pinching the web of a common frog, that, although in the spot actually squeezed, the pigment-cells were deprived of their power of changing, a pale Ping about one-sixteenth of an inch in breadth has gradually formed in its immediate vicinity in the course of the next hour; whence it seems probable that direct irritation tends to excite concentration in the English species as well as in the continental, but that in the former the effect is developed much more slowly, so that it is apt to pass unnoticed. I further, on one occasion, saw *post mortem* concentration greatly accelerated by heat. It is doubtful, however, whether these results are due to direct action upon the pigment-cells; for in the tree frog, as well as in the English kind, the pale tint was not confined to the precise spot operated on, but affected a limited area of surrounding tissue; whence it seems likely that it is developed through the medium of a local nervous apparatus contained in the skin. If this be true, we have no proof that the pigment-cells are capable of being stimulated except by nervous influence, although they are, as we have seen, peculiarly susceptible of suspension of function through the direct operation of irritants upon them.

With regard to the nature of the change experienced by the tissues when temporarily deprived of power by irritants, the primary increase of motion of the cilia, lapsing into quiescence, under the operation of heat, may suggest the idea of exertion followed by exhaustion. But that the state of incapacity is not dependent on previous action, seems clear from the fact that in the pigment-cells it is maintained and aggravated by an irritant continuing in operation after complete suspension of function has been induced, the same kind of effect being still produced upon the tissues which are unable to act as upon healthy parts. As an illustration of this, I may revert to the results of immersion of an amputated limb in aerated water. The carbonic acid, as we have seen, entirely prevents the occurrence of *post mortem* concentration, implying that the powers of the chromatophorous cells are completely suspended by it within a few minutes at most of its first acting on the part; yet, however long the tissues thus paralysed are kept subjected to its influence, they remain without any sign of action. They will, however, recover speedily and completely if soon taken out and exposed to the air, so that the irritating gas may be dissipated; whereas if retained for several hours in the aerated water, they may, indeed, have their powers restored to a certain extent on removal from it, but exhibit only very feeble action. Such facts as these prove conclusively that the tissues may have their functional activity impaired without loss of vitality by the direct action of irritants, independently of any stimulating effects which may be at first produced by them; and also that the influence thus exerted is of an injurious tendency.

The imperceptible transition from suspension of function to loss of vitality displayed by the long-continued operation of carbonic acid upon the pigment-cells is also well illustrated by some of the experiments upon the cilia, especially those with heat and ammonia, which, unless employed with extreme caution, not only permanently arrested the vibratile filaments, but reduced the epithelium-cells to a condition in which they were amenable to the ordinary laws of chemical affinity. All irritants appear to be agents which, if operating with sufficient energy, completely destroy vitality, probably by inducing, through chemical or physical action, an irreparable derangement of the molecular constitution of the tissues. Their essential property, however, is that of causing, when applied somewhat more mildly, a minor degree of disturbance or disorder in the component textures of the body, which are rendered for the time being unfit for discharging their wonted functions, though afterwards, by virtue of their innate powers, capable of spontaneous recovery, the rapidity and completeness of which bears an inverse ratio to the intensity and duration of the previous irritation. Lastly, these same noxious agents, if in a still more gentle form, operate, upon some of the tissues at least, as stimulants, rousing them to increased exertion of their vital functions. How this effect is brought about must, I believe, be only matter of uncertain speculation, so long as the real nature of life in the animal frame remains, as it probably ever will remain to our finite capacities, an impenetrable mystery.

It is an interesting circumstance that, in the experiments with warm water, the cilia, after recovering from the state of quiescence, moved for a while more briskly than they did immediately before the application was made. This increased action cannot be attributed, like the primary acceleration resulting from very gentle warmth, to a mild operation of the irritant; for the epithelium-cells must have been completely cooled down before it commenced. It must therefore be regarded as a true reaction on the part of the tissue, whether dependent on accumulation of vital energy during the period of suspended function, or excited, as by an irritant, by the state of disorder which the warm water had induced, seems uncertain. Considering the number and variety of the functions which direct observation has shown to be suspended by irritants, viz. pigmentary concentration and diffusion, ciliary motion and nervous action, it appears probable that all the vital processes are liable to similar temporary arrest.

Different tissues, however, seem to differ in the facility with which they are affected by irritants. The pigment-cells are very susceptible to their influence, as is indicated by the complete paralysis which we have seen to be produced in them by agencies that give rise to only a minor degree of inflammatory congestion; and also by the circumstance which I have often observed in the web of the frog, that, as in the choroid coat of the human eye, they become absorbed in parts which have been injured, having been deprived of vitality by causes which inflicted on other textures only a recoverable lesion. The epithelium-cells, too, are very sensitive to irritation, exhibiting its results more rapidly than can be accounted for merely by their exposed situation. In those which invest the mucous membrane of the mouth, the cilia with which they are provided furnish the opportunity of which we have availed ourselves, of observing the stage of suspension of function in consequence of very gentle treatment; and though the epidermis does not admit of this, it shows the further stage of loss of vitality by exfoliating after an amount of injury from which the immediately subjacent tissues readily recover. JOHN HUNTER was unquestionably correct in the opinion that the elevation of the cuticle in vesication depends not only on the effusion of serum beneath it, but on a primary separation arising "from a degree of weakness approaching to a kind of death in the connexion between the cuticle and cutis." For I find that in an amputated limb free from blood, although no effusion of serum can occur, the epidermis becomes speedily loosened in a part to which an irritant is applied, as for example, in a web treated with oil of turpentine, whereas it remains elsewhere firmly attached for days if the weather be cool.

The temporary abolition of the normal relations between the blood and the tissues in inflammatory congestion, must be added to the list of instances of suspension of vital properties by irritation. The tissues the healthy state of which seems most likely to be essential to that of the vital fluid, are those contiguous to it, viz. the walls of the blood-vessels; and that these are really deprived of their vital endowments during inflammation, seems implied by the character of the material which is transmitted through them in that condition. For we have seen that the vascular parietes differ, in the state of health, from all ordinary solids in being destitute of any attraction for the fibrine, if not positively repelling it, and that this is probably the cause of the merely serous character of the effusion which takes place in mechanical dropsy depending upon abnormal pressure of the blood within healthy vessels. On the other hand, the exudation of the liquor sanguinis in its integrity, such as occurs in severe inflammation, cannot, I think, be satisfactorily explained by the mere abnormal pressure of the blood produced by dilatation of the arteries and concomitant obstruction in the capillaries; but seems naturally accounted for on the hypothesis that the walls of the vessels, like other tissues, lose, for the time, in inflammation, their vital properties, and, acquiring an attraction for the fibrine like that exercised by ordinary solids, permit it to pass without opposition through their porous parietes.

It may be well to present a brief summary of the principal results arrived at in the present section.

It appears that the various physical and chemical agents which, when operating powerfully, extinguish the life of the constituents of the animal body, produce by a somewhat gentler action a condition bordering upon loss of vitality, but quite distinct from it, in which the tissues are, for the time being, incapacitated for discharging their wonted offices, though retaining the faculty of returning afterwards, by virtue of their own inherent powers, to their former state of activity, provided the irritation have not been too severe or protracted. This suspension of function or temporary abolition of vital energy is the primary lesion in inflammatory congestion; the blood in the vicinity of the disabled tissues assuming the same characters as when in contact with ordinary solid matter, and thus becoming unfit for transmission through the vessels; while the return of the living solids to their usual active state is accompanied by a restoration of the vital fluid to the healthy characters which adapt it for circulation.

Conclusion

It remains to glance at the application of the principles established in the preceding pages to human pathology.

The post mortem appearance which is universally admitted to indicate that the early stages of inflammation have occurred during life, is intense redness, depending essentially not upon peculiar distension of the vessels with blood, but upon abnormal accumulation of the red corpuscles in their minutest ramifications. A beautiful example of this condition, developed idiopathically, was presented by the case of incipient meningitis mentioned in the Introduction, in which the vessels of an affected spot of pia mater were filled with a crimson mass of confusedly compacted corpuscles, exactly as in an area of the frog's web to which mustard has been applied. The derangement of the vital fluid in the human subject being thus closely parallel to that which we have studied in the batrachian reptile, we can hardly doubt that in the former, as in the latter, the living solids are in a state of more or less complete suspension of functional activity during inflammatory congestion. This view is supported by the effusion of liquor sanguinis in its integrity in the more advanced stages of the disease in man, and by the speedy coagulation of fibrine upon inflamed serous surfaces, or in the interior of vessels affected with arteritis or phlebitis. For these circumstances, as has been before remarked, appear to indicate that the tissues are for the time being reduced still more towards the condition of ordinary solid matter. These arguments, derived from the appearances of the blood, are further corroborated by the immediate transition which is apt to occur from intense human inflammation to gangrene.

But a comprehensive and complete account of the inflammatory process must embrace not merely the state to which the tissues are brought when the disease is fairly established, but also the causes which lead to it.

Inflammation is sometimes brought about in man in a way strictly analogous to that in which we induce it in the web of the frog's foot, viz, by the immediate operation of some noxious agent from without, as when boiling water is poured upon the skin. One peculiarity connected with such cases, as compared with those which are of idiopathic origin, is the great rapidity with which the various stages of the disorder are often developed. This, however, is the natural consequence of the direct manner in which the prejudicial influence is exerted upon the tissues; the inflammatory phenomena supervening more speedily in proportion to the energy of the irritant. This principle is well illustrated by the effects of mechanical violence upon the human integument. A moderate degree of pressure applied continuously gives rise, during the first few hours, to nothing more than inflammatory congestion, which disappears soon after the pressure has been removed, as seen in the red mark produced upon the forehead by a tightly fitting hat. But if such treatment be continued for a considerably longer period, vesication mill result, as when apparatus employed for the treatment of fractures is applied too firmly for many hours together over a bony prominence. The same effect which is thus slowly developed under a moderate degree of mechanical irritation, may, however, be induced very rapidly through the same agency in a more intense form, as is shown by the bulla: which are often observed in surgical practice very soon after the infliction of a severe contusion. Here the source of irritation being no longer in operation, there is no blush of redness in the vicinity dependent upon arterial dilatation, and hence such cases are often supposed to have nothing in common with inflammation; and I have known these vesicles mistaken for evidence of gangrene, so as to lead to unnecessary amputation. The suddenness with which inflammatory aedema arises in consequence of the bites or stings of venomous reptiles is explicable on the same principle. The poison appears to diffuse itself among the tissues so as to operate directly upon them, and when extremely virulent, kills them outright; but when less potent, produces merely a temporary though rapid prostration of their vital energies with consequent inflammatory effusion. Again, the congestion of the lungs, which comes on so quickly in asphyxia, has been before alluded to, as probably the result of the sedative influence which, from experiments upon the frog, we are led to believe must be produced upon the pulmonary tissue by the abnormal amount of carbonic acid in the air-cells.

In the class of cases hitherto considered, the derangement of the part, and the causes which lead to it, being both, to a considerable extent, understood, the disease may, 1 think, be regarded as in so far satisfactorily explained. But one important lesson taught by the results of this investigation is, that it is necessary to draw a broad line of demarcation between inflammation produced by direct irritation, and that which is developed indirectly through the medium of the nervous system, whether in the immediate vicinity of a source of irritation, as around a tight stitch in the skin, or a thorn in the finger, or at a distance from the disturbing cause, as when the kidneys are affected in consequence of the passing of a bougie, or the lungs through exposure of the feet to cold. Nothing can better illustrate the importance of this distinction, than what takes place in a recent wound. In consequence of the injury inflicted by the knife, together with the subsequent manipulation and exposure, the tissues, in a thin layer at the cut surface, are thrown into that condition which leads to effusion of liquor sanguinis, the fibrine of which, speedily coagulating, remains to constitute the bond of primary union, while the serum trickling away between the lips of the wound produces the discharge which soaks the dressing during the first twenty-four hours. But neither during the exudation of the lymph in such a case, nor during its subsequent organization, is there necessarily any inflammation induced in the lips of the wound through the nervous system; and if this complication does occur, it interferes with the healing process in a degree proportioned to its intensity. In other words, while a certain amount of inflammation as caused by direct irritation is essential to primary union, any degree of it as induced indirectly is both unnecessary and injurious.

The question how inflammation is developed through the medium of the nervous system, possesses a high degree of interest, in consequence of its bearing upon the manner in which counter-irritation operates therapeutically. In the integument, where we have the opportunity of seeing the affected part, the first indication of the supervention of inflammatory disorder around a centre of irritation is a blush of redness, which, as before shown, consists, in the first instance, of mere dilatation of the arteries with rapid flow of blood through the capillaries. It is quite conceivable that arterial dilatation, carried to an extreme degree along with powerful action of the heart?, may so increase the tension upon the tissues as to impair their powers gradually by mechanical irritation, just as the frontal integument is affected by long-continued gentle pressure from without, as above alluded to; for we know that when inflammation does exist, mere increase of tension upon the blood in the vessels will greatly aggravate the disorder, as when an inflamed foot is kept in a dependent posture. Supposing this to be the whole mechanism of the disease, its origin would be sufficiently intelligible;

for we have seen that vascular dilatation caused by irritation operating through the medium of the nervous system appears to depend on a depressing influence produced by excessive action of the afferent nerves upon the ganglia which preside over the arterial contractions. There are, however, some circumstances, such as the dryness of the nostril which may exist in the early stages of coryza, and sudden suppression of urine in consequence of urethral irritation in cases where renal congestion becomes ultimately established, which seem to indicate that other functions as well as arterial contraction may be primarily arrested by nervous agency in the early stages of inflammation. The study of the pigmentary system of the frog has afforded proof that other tissues besides muscular fibre are under the control of the nerves, and it seems not unlikely that gland-cells or other forms of tissue may, like nerve-cells, be reduced to a state of inactivity by excessive nervous action; and thus we seem to have a clue to comprehending what at first appears anomalous, that prostration of the vital energies of the part actually inflamed may be brought about by unusually great activity in the parts of the nervous system specially concerned with it. This, however, is a wide subject, which requires further investigation. But in the mean time we may, I think, consider as satisfactorily established the fundamental principle, that whenever inflammatory congestion, or, in other words, that disturbance of the circulation which is truly characteristic of inflammation, exists in any degree, the tissues of the affected part have experienced to a proportionate extent a temporary impairment of functional activity or vital energy.